The Essentials of Pouch Care Nursing

EDITED BY

JULIA WILLIAMS MEd, BSc(HONS), RGN, DIPD/N

Lecturer in Gastro-intestinal Nursing,
St Mark's Hospital, Harrow

W
WHURR PUBLISHERS
LONDON AND PHILADELPHIA

© 2002 Whurr Publishers Ltd
First published 2002
by Whurr Publishers Ltd
19b Compton Terrace
London N1 2UN England and
325 Chestnut Street, Philadelphia PA 19106 USA

British Library Cataloguing in Publication Data

A catalogue record for this book
is available from the British Library.

ISBN 1 86156 221 7

Printed and bound in the UK by Athenaeum Press Ltd,
Gateshead, Tyne & Wear.

Contents

Foreword

The introduction of the ileal reservoir by Kock in the late 1960s to improve quality of life for the ileostomist was the start of a long development in intestinal surgery. Soon afterwards, restorative proctocolectomy with ileoanal reservoir was designed by Parks in order to avoid ileostomy altogether. Subsequently, the use of the colonic reservoir by Lazorthes aimed to improve bowel function in patients with low anterior resection. Thus, pouch surgery has been applied to inflammatory bowel disease, rectal cancer and familial adenomatous polyposis, becoming an important part of specialist colorectal surgery.

Pouches have much to do with quality of life, and this to a degree depends on the subjective perception of the patient. The discussion of indications, including counselling, is thus a vital element of achieving an optimum result. Following surgery, the patient requires help in dealing with normal recovery – even more so in the event of complications. Long-term follow-up and continued support after leaving hospital are therefore necessary. It is with these aspects of care that specialist nurses can help in a way that doctors cannot easily do. They have a different perspective on the patient's dilemma of choice of procedure and on the consideration of possible disadvantages. In addition, they can, by their accessibility, more readily offer continuity of care and advice.

Decision-making, preparation for surgery, the intermediate postoperative course and longer-term outcomes all come within the ambit of this excellent book. The vast amount of information available on pouches has been summarised in various chapters to enable a rapid and easy access to important issues, both surgical and nursing. *The Essentials of Pouch Nursing* is the first book of its kind. It fills an educational gap and will be essential reading for any health-care professional with an interest in colorectal reconstructive surgery. It deals with all the diseases amenable to pouch formation, as well as with various techniques and aftercare, in a highly practical manner.

Professor R. John Nicholls
St Mark's Hospital, Harrow
July 2001

Contributors

Pat Coldicutt BA(Hons) RGN RSCN DPSN Clinical Nurse Specialist – Stoma Care, Alder Hey Children's Hospital, Liverpool

Gail Fitzpatrick RGN RSCN Clinical Nurse Specialist – Stoma Care, The Birmingham Children's Hospital NHS Trust, Birmingham

Alastair Forbes BSc MD FRCP Consultant Physician, North West London Hospitals Trust, St Mark's Hospital, Harrow, Middlesex

Darren Gold MSc FRCS(Gen) Senior Registrar, North West London Hospitals Trust, St Mark's Hospital, Harrow, Middlesex

Peter Hawley MS FRCS Consultant Surgeon, The London Clinic, Harley Street, London

Rachel Leaver BSc(Hons) RGN Clinical Nurse Specialist – Continent Urinary Diversions, UCL Hospitals NHS Trust, St. Peter's Hospital, London

Kay Neale MSc SRN Registrar, The Polyposis Registry, North West London Hospitals Trust, St. Mark's Hospital, Harrow, Middlesex.

R. John Nicholls MA Mchir FRCS FRCPS(Glas) Consultant Surgeon, Clinical Director, North West London Hospitals Trust, St Mark's Hospital, Harrow, Middlesex

John Northover MS FRCS Consultant Surgeon, North West London Hospitals Trust, St Mark's Hospital, Harrow, Middlesex

Morag Pearson BSc (Hons), SRD Senior Dietician, North West London Hospitals Trust, St Mark's Hospital, Harrow, Middlesex

Robin Phillips MS FRCS Consultant Surgeon and Dean, St Mark's Academic Institute, North West London Hospitals Trust, St Mark's Hospital, Harrow, Middlesex

Mave Salter MSc BSc(Hons) RGN BNDN(Cert) CertEdRNT ENB
    216 CSCT Clinical Nurse Specialist, The Royal Marsden
    Hospital NHS Trust, Sutton, Surrey
Claire Taylor MSc BSc RGN Colorectal Macmillan Nurse Special-
    ist, North West London Hospitals Trust, St Mark's Hospital,
    Harrow, Middlesex.
Julia Williams MEd BSc(Hons) RGN Dip DN Lecturer in
    Gastro-intestinal Nursing, North West London Hospitals Trust,
    St Mark's Hospital, Harrow, Middlesex

Acknowledgements

I would like to thank all those who contributed a chapter to this book.

Special thanks go to my colleagues within the Stoma Care Department, St Mark's Hospital, particularly Professor R. John Nicholls, for supporting me throughout this project. I am also grateful to Dansac Ltd for making the vision become true.

Finally, sincere thanks go to my family and friends for their continued support and encouragement.

dansac O

Dansac Limited are proud to have been invited to support Julia Williams with this very important publication.

Dansac Limited believes that as a leading manufacturer within the stoma care market, we have a responsibility to health-care professionals to help provide continuing education and support wherever appropriate.

We are pleased to have provided financial support for this book, and to have donated a copy to each Stoma Care Department within the UK.

CHAPTER 1

Medical aspects of ulcerative colitis

ALASTAIR FORBES

Ulcerative colitis is one of the two principal forms of inflammatory bowel disease and is somewhat more common than Crohn's disease. Although some aspects of this discussion apply equally to Crohn's disease, it should be assumed that ulcerative colitis is under consideration unless this is otherwise specified.

Epidemiology

Ulcerative colitis affects men and women at a similar rate and with a similar severity. There is a steady annual incidence of around 7 per 100,000 population, the highest figures being seen in regions most distant from the equator. The peak times for first presentation and for relapses are in the early spring and autumn/winter, with a relative lack of clinical events in the late spring and summer months: December is almost twice as problematic as May.

Aetiology and pathogenesis

The aetiology and pathogenesis of ulcerative colitis have a limited bearing on clinical practice, but it is hoped that the following will aid an understanding of the disease process and of the mechanisms by which therapeutic agents act. It should also help to provide answers to some of the questions asked by patients about their disease.

In ulcerative colitis, there are almost certainly both inherited factors and environmental influences acting together.

1

Genetics of ulcerative colitis

The risk of a sufferer's sibling, parent or child being affected lies at between 1 in 15 and 1 in 10, which is about 50 times the risk in the general population. However, in only around 1 out of 10 pairs of even identical twins do both members develop ulcerative colitis. Within families, colitis seems to occur at a younger age in successive generations.

Links with the HLA tissue-typing antigens have been sought. Certain HLA DR2 antigens are over-represented (being seen in around 40% of colitics compared with about 20% of control populations) and are also associated with a higher frequency of total colitis and need for surgery. In addition to the HLA sites on chromosome 6, there are putative genes coding for ulcerative colitis on chromosomes 2, 3, 7 and 12.

A circulating antibody to a neutrophil cytoplasmic antigen is rarely seen other than in colitis, its presence being partly genetically determined. Antibody levels do not reflect disease activity but do tend to fall slowly after colectomy.

The striking demarcation of the upper limit of ulcerative colitis (see below) may also be genetically determined via a variance in the anatomy of the marginal artery, a normally small branch of the inferior mesenteric artery. This hypothesis, however, remains controversial.

Infection as the cause of inflammatory bowel disease

Although most attention to infection as a possible cause of inflammatory bowel disease has focused on Crohn's disease, there is also evidence relevant to ulcerative colitis. The seasonal variation in clinical activity has already been referred to, and patients often link gastrointestinal infections to the onset or relapse of their colitis.

Hydrogen sulphide, a product of sulphate-reducing bacteria, is specifically implicated. Many colitis patients describe offensive flatus, and although it is for obvious reasons difficult to perform studies of flatus, data do exist. Colitis patients produce up to four times as much hydrogen sulphide as normal people. This is not only unpleasant, but also toxic, with an effect in animals similar to that of cyanide.

There may also be an immune response to normal intestinal organisms, with a significant level of circulating antibodies to a variety of their antigens. Purified bacterial components can produce intestinal inflammation, but there is little evidence that ulcerative colitis is truly an autoimmune disease.

In animal models of inflammatory bowel disease, it is striking that bacteria are almost always involved in addition to the specific stimulus employed. Few animals spontaneously develop a disease at all like colitis, an endangered monkey, the cotton-top tamarin, being an exception. Tamarin colitis is very similar to ulcerative colitis, including the propensity for colorectal carcinoma to develop; the disease seems only to affect animals held in captivity.

Non-steroidal anti-inflammatory drugs

Non-steroidal anti-inflammatory drugs may be implicated in the causation of some cases of inflammatory bowel disease. These drugs can certainly cause colonic inflammation, watery diarrhoea and chronic blood loss. Even if not causative, they tend to exaggerate symptoms in many (if not most) patients with colitis. They may also be responsible for a high proportion of cases of acute self-limiting colitis.

Smoking and colitis

Smoking is an intriguing environmental factor in the context of inflammatory bowel disease. It definitely contributes adversely to all aspects of Crohn's disease but appears in some way protective in ulcerative colitis. Smoking is less common in ulcerative colitis patients than in healthy controls, the highest frequency of the disease being found in ex-smokers. It also influences the ileo-anal pouch, pouchitis being less common in current smokers. The reason(s) for this remain speculative, but a disruption of mucus production and of protective barrier function is probably important. Nicotine may also be helpful, and this has led to several trials of its use.

Appendicectomy

For reasons that are not clear, previous appendicectomy is protective against, or is associated with a protective factor against, ulcerative colitis. Patients with colitis are only about a twentieth as likely to have had their appendix removed as are age-matched controls.

Diet as an aetiological factor

Although diet is almost certainly important in Crohn's disease, and patients are always concerned to explore a link in ulcerative colitis, there is no clear association, other than in Japanese patients in whom the consumption of a Western-type diet is associated with the disease. Clearly, diet is not an independent risk factor here.

Clinical presentation and investigation

Ulcerative colitis is usually responsible for diarrhoea and rectal bleeding. Less often, there is weight loss, anorexia and fatigue. When there is only a short history, gastrointestinal infection will be the most probable alternative diagnosis. General examination usually contributes little; although perianal disease is more typical of Crohn's disease, some changes are seen in a minority (up to 10%) of patients with ulcerative colitis.

Oral aphthous ulcers are common in the general population but are over-represented in groups of patients with inflammatory bowel disease. They can be troublesome and may need specific treatment with topical steroids to achieve their resolution.

Investigation

At sigmoidoscopy, the rectum is almost always obviously involved in ulcerative colitis. There is a loss of the normal vascular pattern, confluent erythema and, to a greater or lesser degree, ulceration, the latter two being continuous. That is to say, the disease is present distally and extends proximally without uninvolved colon between the abnormal areas.

Investigation will typically commence with routine laboratory tests such as a full blood count and serum biochemistry. These will rarely contribute to the diagnostic process itself, except where there is uncertainty over whether the patient has atypical functional bowel disease (effectively excluded by an elevated platelet count, a low haemoglobin level or low albumin, for example). Blood tests assessing the degree of inflammation, including the C-reactive protein (CRP) level and the erythrocyte sedimentation rate, are also used. These, however, have only modest reliability.

Differential diagnosis

The differential diagnosis of ulcerative colitis includes infection, non-steroidal drug-related colitis and acute self-limiting colitis. The most likely organisms are all are fairly readily identified (or excluded) by a conventional laboratory examination of the stools. 'Pseudo-membranous colitis', arising from *Clostridium difficile* infection should be sought, by culture and by examination for the cytotoxin, especially if the patient has recently been exposed to antibiotics. The patient with ulcerative colitis may also present because of a superimposed gastrointestinal infection.

In the patient presenting without acute dysenteric symptoms, the differential diagnosis includes colorectal carcinoma, ischaemic colitis and radiation enteritis.

Up to a third of patients with predominantly distal colitis may, despite a history of diarrhoea, prove to be constipated on abdominal palpation. A distinction from functional bowel disorders such as irritable bowel syndrome is usually obvious because of the presence of bleeding in colitis.

Barium enema and other imaging

The double-contrast enema using both air and barium has almost completely superseded the single-contrast examination, but the unprepared ('instant') enema is still helpful in the evaluation of acute colitis (Figure 1.1). In early or mild colitis, the only abnormality may be a granularity of the mucosa, but the changes will be continuous from the rectum upwards. The so-called 'hose-pipe' colon is now rarely seen but when present strongly supports the diagnosis of chronic ulcerative colitis.

Computed tomography scanning with computer reconstruction to generate 'virtual colonoscopy' is very impressive as a technological feat, but is not yet as sensitive as colonoscopy. In radio labelled white cell scanning, the patients' own leukocytes are labelled and returned to the circulation. These migrate to areas of inflammation and hence provide a relatively non-invasive definition of the extent of disease in colitis.

Colonoscopy

While there is certainly a place for the barium enema and the other options, none is yet as sensitive as colonoscopy, and none of the

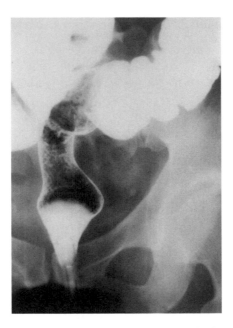

Figure 1.1 Barium enema showing superficial ulceration in the rectum but normal appearances more proximally in a patient with ulcerative colitis.

others permits biopsy samples to be obtained. At colonoscopy, the features are essentially those already described for sigmoidoscopy. The proximal limit of ulcerative colitis is often very clearly demarcated, and the small bowel is never involved (Figures 1.2 and 1.3).

There may be (post-inflammatory) polyps at sites of past inflammation, which can develop into long, interlinked lesions with mucosal bridging. Pseudopolyps, which represent islands of normal or regenerative mucosa, occur only when there is marked active inflammation.

Histology

A firm diagnosis of ulcerative colitis should not be made without histological support. The histological changes are confined to the mucosa and submucosa. There will typically be an acute inflammatory reaction with neutrophils, crypt abscesses and goblet cells depleted of mucus. With time, architectural changes develop. Irregular, short and excessively branched crypts develop. These features are more conclusive in the distinction from acute infective colitis or self-limiting colitis (see Figure 1.2).

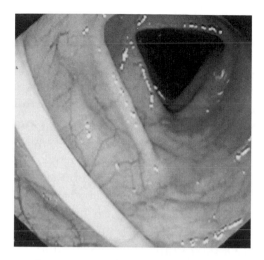

Figure 1.2 Colonoscopic appearance of normal transverse colon in a patient with left-sided colitis (see Plate 1).

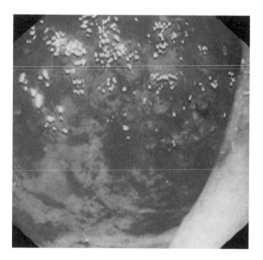

Figure 1.3 Active ulcerative colitis in sigmoid colon (same patient as above) (see Plate 2).

Clinical course and natural history of ulcerative colitis

The clinical course of colitis is not easily predicted, but the extent of colonic involvement is a guide to the future risk of colorectal carcinoma. At any one time, about 50% of patients with colitis are in full remission, but most remain prone to intermittent relapses. Activity in any given year predicts a 70–80% risk of activity in the following year. The cumulative risk of colectomy varies from one centre to another, being partly dependent on the proportion of patients with extensive colitis seen, but it is typically around 1 in 5 at 10 years and nearer 1 in 3 on a lifetime basis.

Most patients with colitis can pursue a normal working life. The risk of relapse probably gradually diminishes with increasing age.

Frequency and significance of proximal extension of distal colitis

Ulcerative colitis is a distal disease with variable proximal extension. Because the proportion of the colon involved has a bearing on the risk of colonic carcinoma, it is used to modify the intensity of hospital follow-up. The colitis may, however, advance proximally with time. In about a quarter of those with initially limited disease, there is a progression to extensive disease by 10 years. Occasional re-evaluation is therefore appropriate.

Psychological and other clinical aspects of ulcerative colitis

It is not unusual for patients with well-established colitis to present with symptoms that sound more functional, investigations such as CRP level being normal. Perhaps as many as a fifth of all patients have irritable bowel syndrome superimposed on the colitis. This can present quite awkward management decisions.

The patient with ulcerative colitis has a chronic and often debilitating disease that can only be cured by radical surgery, which itself leaves variable long-term sequelae. The symptoms of the disease are unpleasant and are not considered ones for 'polite conversation'. It is inevitable therefore that psychological morbidity runs alongside the organic physical disease. No one now would seriously maintain that colitis is caused by psychological disease, but there can be little doubt that psychological factors can be very important, presumably contributing to the functional symptoms described above. The unpredictability of colitis is itself a major cause of anxiety and stress, especially when faecal incontinence is or has ever been a problem.

Given time, patients will often be remarkably candid about the influence of stress and emotional issues on their intestinal symptoms, appearing to find such a discussion therapeutically valuable. They may also be greatly helped by the use of low doses of constipating agents such as loperamide to help them through times of predictable stress. There does not seem to be any risk from this as long as the patient knows to discontinue the drug if true constipation develops or if abdominal discomfort occurs.

Quality of life in colitis

It is obvious that colitis has an adverse impact on the patient's quality of life, the creation and success of patient support groups, such as the National Association for Colitis and Crohn's Disease in Britain, having been partly a response to this. Many useful information leaflets, and practical aids such as the 'Can't wait' card (aiding urgent toilet access) (Figure 1.4), have been produced, in addition to counselling services and informal support. Steps have also been taken to offset discrimination in the workplace and with respect to life insurance.

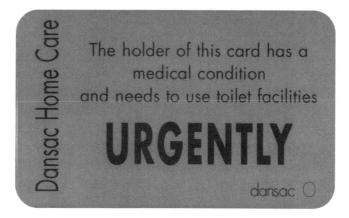

Figure 1.4 'Can't wait' card.

Causes of death in ulcerative colitis

Even allowing for colorectal carcinoma, colitis has little overall effect on mortality. There is a reduced life expectancy, but at 20 years it is still at least 90–95% that of controls, even in those with extensive colitis. The standardized mortality ratio of around 1.35 reflects an overall threefold increase in the number of colorectal carcinoma deaths and excess deaths from sclerosing cholangitis.

Medical therapy

Corticosteroids and the 5-aminosalicylate (5-ASA) drugs (sulphasalazine and its successors) still constitute the mainstay of drug therapy, azathioprine being established for resistant disease. The remitting and relapsing course of colitis, and the substantial rate of spontaneous improvement whatever therapeutic endeavours are employed, makes it crucial that any new measures should be compared with established treatments in randomized, blind, controlled trials. Previous placebo-controlled trials indicate that spontaneous improvement and an apparently full remission may reasonably be expected in around 30% and 10% of exacerbations respectively.

Steroids

Corticosteroids (usually prednisolone or hydrocortisone) provide a rapid and effective relief of symptoms in acute exacerbations, albeit not always accompanied by a full remission. There is little difference between hydrocortisone and prednisolone when equivalent doses are compared (4 mg methylprednisolone: 5 mg prednisolone: 25 mg hydrocortisone). Intravenous therapy is probably more potent than oral treatment in resistant cases.

Typical regimes for moderate to severe colitis comprise oral prednisolone 0.5–1.0 mg per kilogram body weight, with a suggested minimum of 30 mg daily. There are no good data to determine how long this dose should be maintained, and most gastroenterologists commence a fairly brisk reduction once the response begins in order to avoid unnecessary toxicity. A typical regime is 7 days at the starting dose, reducing thereafter by 5 mg per week until weaning is complete.

Steroids are ineffective in maintaining remission and cause significant long-term side-effects, so they should be withdrawn once the acute episode has settled. Unfortunately, a few patients do become steroid dependent, fostering an interest in new, less toxic, steroids. Delayed-release oral budesonide fits this description and compares reasonably well with prednisolone in efficacy, having notably less toxicity. Budesonide enemas are therapeutically equivalent to hydro-cortisone and prednisolone in acute distal colitis, but they are less readily absorbed and cause less adrenal suppression. If long-term steroid use is really necessary, this drug should perhaps now be chosen.

Aminosalicylates

Sulphasalazine has been used in the treatment of ulcerative colitis since the early 1950s, proving effective in acute colitis and in the maintenance of remission. A reduction in the annual relapse rate from approximately 70% in the untreated to around 25% in those taking the drug is typical. Up to 15% of individuals are intolerant of the sulphapyridine component of sulphasalazine, but most of its therapeutic benefit results from the 5-ASA (or mesalazine) molecule. Oral 5-ASA is ineffective because it is absorbed and metabolized too proximally; alternative formulations of 5-ASA have therefore been developed. There is also no problem with oligospermia with the newer agents.

In 1999, six 5-ASA preparations were commercially available in Europe. Asacol is 5-ASA coated with a resin, which releases the drug when the pH is above 7.0, this typically occurring in the region of the caecum and ascending colon. The resin coat of Claversal and Salofalk dissolves a little more proximally. Pentasa has microgran-ules of 5-ASA in a semi-permeable membrane, its 5-ASA being steadily released throughout the intestine. Olsalazine has two mole-cules of 5-ASA linked by a bond that is broken by the same colonic bacterial enzymes that activate sulphasalazine. A potential advan-tage of olsalazine over other 5-ASA preparations is limited by an osmotic diarrhoea provoked by the drug, which affects up to 10% of patients but may be minimized by taking the drug with food. Balsalazide has a bond linking 5-ASA to an inert carrier and is handled like olsalazine.

The difference between all these 5-ASA agents is relatively minor, all appearing to be superior to sulphasalazine, although olsalazine and balsalazide may have the edge in more distal disease. Around

60% of patients with moderately active colitis will respond to 5-ASA therapy alone. There are strong suggestions that regular and long-term 5-ASA use not only prolongs the relapse-free interval survival, but also helps to reduce the risk of colonic neoplasia. Patients in prolonged remission nevertheless usually seek to stop maintenance therapy – or simply stop it. Aside from the issue of cancer risk, this becomes increasingly reasonable the longer the patient is from the last relapse.

The 5-ASA drugs are very occasionally responsible for renal toxicity via an interstitial nephritis, which may lead to end-stage renal failure. It is probably an idiosyncratic, dose-independent effect and occurs with all formulations including sulphasalazine, although it is recorded more often with pH delivery systems. A periodic assessment of renal function (perhaps every 6 months) is therefore wise as early changes are probably not progressive even if they are not fully reversible. 5-ASA preparations are themselves rarely the cause of an exacerbation of the colitis, the associated worsening of the underlying disease potentially leading to confusion until the correct interpretation has been reached.

Topical 5-ASA is firmly established in the treatment of active proctitis and distal colitis, typically with a response rate in excess of 70% over 3–6 weeks. The results are at least as good as, and probably better than, those of topical steroids and oral 5-ASA. In the UK, topical steroids are, however, a great deal cheaper and will probably remain the first choice in most units. Topical steroids and 5-ASA preparations may also usefully be combined. Patients almost always prefer foams to liquid enemas, but suppositories are quite often sufficient in the most distal disease, an adequate amount being delivered by a single daily 1 g dose of 5-ASA.

Immunosuppressant therapy

Immunosuppressant drugs are valuable in refractory colitis but have limited efficacy and significant toxicity. Trials of other immunomodulatory are also underway.

Azathioprine

Azathioprine and 6-mercaptopurine inhibit the synthesis of DNA and RNA. They are effective in refractory ulcerative colitis but work slowly, so it can be 3 months before the full benefit is seen. Approximately two-thirds of patients will both tolerate and respond to the drugs.

Most side-effects are relatively trivial, but pancreatitis, hepatitis and hypersensitivity reactions do occur. Absorbed azathioprine is almost entirely metabolized to 6-mercaptopurine and then to 6-methylmercaptopurine. The enzyme responsible for this second step (thiopurine methyltransferase) is genetically deficient in many otherwise normal people, who are, as a result, at higher risk of bone marrow suppression. Unfortunately, it is not routinely possible to test the level of the enzyme, so continuing caution must be adopted.

The bone marrow suppression is dose related and reversible. It usually occurs in the first 6 months of treatment but can occur much later, this danger therefore necessitating a regular 4–6 weekly monitoring of the white blood cell count while therapy continues.

Ciclosporin

Ciclosporin is a potent immunosuppressant widely used in transplant recipients. A continuous infusion of 4 mg/kg per day yields a substantial advantage over high-dose steroids alone in about 60% of unresponsive patients with fulminant colitis (see below). This improvement seems to be maintained in about half of those who respond initially.

There is a real danger of death from overwhelming immunosuppression, and of other serious side-effects, including renal failure and grand mal fits, which may potentially outweigh the advantages of a lower colectomy rate. It is not yet clear whether ciclosporin has a role in maintenance or in the chronically steroid-dependent patient.

Methotrexate

Methotrexate has immunosuppressive and anti-inflammatory properties, hence its use in psoriasis and rheumatoid arthritis. Although there is good evidence that it can be effective in Crohn's disease, there are no satisfactory data to support its use in ulcerative colitis.

Antibiotics for the specific treatment of ulcerative colitis

Antibiotics have an obvious role in the management of the infective complications of colitis, but it has also been suggested that they might have a specific effect on the underlying disease process. Evidence for this is slim, but there are suggestions that tobramycin, co-amoxiclav and ciprofloxacin may have a useful effect.

Nutrition as specific treatment of ulcerative colitis

Nutritional intervention is crucial in malnourished patients, but, unlike the situation in Crohn's disease, in which it may have value as a primary therapy, there is no evidence that this applies to ulcerative colitis. Many patients nevertheless find that dietary changes have a major impact on their symptoms, possibly because of a modification of the colonic bacterial flora.

An increased intake of fish oil may help by limiting thromboxane and prostaglandin formation, and a high-fibre intake provides more colonic free fatty acids, which are important colonocyte nutrients. It is difficult to give constructive advice that will be of general value, but it is worth encouraging patients to make their own explorations into dietary manipulation. A reduction in the consumption of milk products may also be helpful.

Tumour necrosis factor and other cytokines

The inflammatory cytokines contribute to the inflammatory response in inflammatory bowel disease, and there has been a huge investment in their manipulation in Crohn's disease, with encouraging results. There has, however, been much less attention paid to their role in ulcerative colitis, although preliminary data suggest that intravenous antibodies to tumour necrosis factor, and topical interleukin-10, may also have a place in colitis therapy.

Heparin therapy for colitis

Heparin is best known as an anticoagulant but also has anti-inflammatory properties. Following cases in which heparin, given for incidental deep venous thromboses, has appeared to be effective in problematic ulcerative colitis, there is an expanding world literature favouring full heparinization as a treatment for colitis. Controlled data are as yet lacking, but there are laboratory grounds for believing that the response is explicable on scientific grounds through effects on leukocyte adhesion and mucosal repair in a context in which the body's endogenous heparin equivalent is deficient.

Nicotine

Intermittent smokers and those who restart after a period of abstinence often record an improvement in their ulcerative colitis symptoms. Although it is clearly not the only constituent of cigarette smoke, nicotine has been assessed as a potential therapeutic agent. Nicotine patches have shown some beneficial effect in active ulcerative colitis (similar in degree to the benefit expected from 5-ASA therapy), but side-effects limit their widespread use. Newer approaches in which nicotine is delivered in a non-absorbed form to the distal bowel are showing more promise. Curiously, there is no benefit from maintenance use. The evidence in favour of smoking (as opposed to nicotine administration alone) is insufficient to warrant its recommendation to ulcerative colitis patients, given its other potentially fatal consequences.

Acute severe or fulminant colitis

Acute severe or fulminant colitis remains an important clinical problem and is still responsible for major morbidity and occasional deaths. In many respects, its medical management is simple, but the necessity and timing of surgery can remain difficult to judge.

Fulminant colitis is defined by the combination of frequent bloody diarrhoea with evidence of systemic illness in the form of tachycardia, pyrexia, anaemia, a low albumin level and so on. Its mortality has fallen substantially since the middle of the twentieth century, from around 50% before the introduction of steroids in the early 1950s, to around 1.5% in most centres today. This reduction has not, however, been the result of single critical changes in practice, as even steroids brought the mortality down to only around 30%. The improvement almost certainly reflects earlier diagnosis, better medical and perioperative care (including safer anaesthesia) and, possibly most importantly, the greater sharing of management between physicians and surgeons.

This cooperation unfortunately appears to function least well in centres with the least experience of life-threatening colitis. Any patient sick enough to warrant admission for ulcerative colitis really also warrants referral to both medical and surgical gastroenterologists. This practice makes joint planning easier and eliminates the surgeons' concerns that some patients are referred too late, as well as the physicians' frustrations, when having managed the patient actively for some days and reached the conclusion that surgery is inevitable, the surgeon chooses to observe for a further period while becoming familiar with the patient.

There is rarely a substantial differential diagnosis when the patient is already known to have ulcerative colitis, but it can be the first evidence of colitis, and in the known colitic, as well as in new cases, it is essential to exclude infective causes and, perhaps especially, superimposed *Clostridium difficile* infection. The immediate management of fulminant colitis includes bed-rest and intravenous steroids, with parenteral fluids and blood if necessary. A regime based on prednisolone 1 mg/kg or hydrocortisone 5 mg/kg is appropriate. The response to steroid therapy can be anticipated in about two-thirds of these patients. Bowel rest from intravenous nutrition does not appear to offer any advantage.

Urgent surgery is almost always indicated in fulminant colitis if complications arise. It is mandatory in the event of perforation and virtually so in major haemorrhage (the transfusion of more than 6 units or the daily administration of blood). Surgery should naturally follow full resuscitative measures and should be performed by an experienced colorectal surgeon.

Toxic megacolon

Toxic megacolon complicates no more than 10% of cases with fulminant colitis, but it is the major indication for surgery in around 25% of urgent cases. The condition is readily defined from the diameter of the colon or caecum on a plain abdominal radiograph (Figure 1.5). It is usually easiest to identify in the transverse colon, where a diameter in excess of 5.5 cm is considered diagnostic in the context of acute colitis (Figure 1.5). The predominance of this site simply reflects the colonic anatomy, as this is generally the least dependent part of the colon when the patient lies supine and is therefore gas-filled and most easily visualized. A caecal diameter of more than 9 cm has an identical significance.

Many gastroenterologists and most surgeons consider megacolon to be an absolute indication for colectomy. This is a safe but perhaps unnecessarily aggressive strategy. It is probably reasonable to permit 24 hours of medical therapy in a patient who presents untreated with

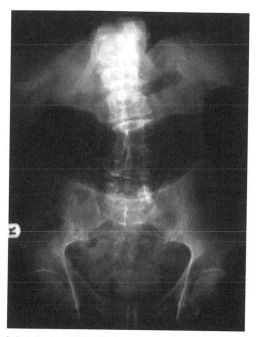

Figure 1.5 Plain abdominal radiograph in a patient with fulminant ulcerative colitis; the diameter of the transverse colon is greatly enlarged, and without urgent surgery there is a major risk of perforation.

megacolon, but megacolon developing during therapy or persisting for more than 24 hours despite therapy should lead to colectomy. Both the use of a rectal tube and rolling or other positional changes of the patient may help in deflation of the bowel.

All forms of medical therapy for megacolon may, however, be considered to be temporizing manoeuvres as around 50% of patients so treated come to colectomy within a year. Equally, some of these are able to have elective surgery, with its obvious advantages relative to emergency resection. It should be remembered that evidence of serious complications such as perforation and faecal peritonitis can be masked by the high doses of steroids being used. A low threshold for surgical intervention should thus be maintained.

Prognostic markers

Predictors of the failure of medical therapy once the major complications have been sought and excluded reflect evidence of disease severity and involvement of the full thickness of the colon. The stool frequency and the CRP level on day 3 are particularly helpfully associated with the final outcome, such that the huge majority of those who still have more than eight stools a day, or a CRP level still greater than 45 mg/l, will require colectomy.

In addition to toxic megacolon, there are other abnormalities discernible from the plain abdominal radiograph that are predictive of a poor outcome. The presence of mucosal islands along the length of the colon indicates a virtually complete loss of the mucosal surface, the beginnings of full-thickness damage to the bowel and a very high risk of later perforation if colectomy is not undertaken. These islands are in fact the last remaining regions of relatively preserved mucosa. The presence of multiple dilated loops of small bowel is similarly disconcerting.

Assessment

A suggested framework of clinical and investigatory monitoring is given in Table 1.1. Most of the elements are standard observations, but it is surprisingly informative to collect the various items onto a single 'colitis observations proforma'. Although there is an implicit benefit in a daily assessment of the fulminant colitic by a senior clinician, who will often be able to provide a reliable overall assessment from clinical review alone, the global assessments made by the well-supported nurse or junior doctor using the proforma are rarely different. The measurement of abdominal girth is notoriously irreproducible and is not recommended.

Surgery for fulminant colitis

Early surgery should be considered for fulminant colitis if any complication develops or if there is an overall deterioration despite appropriate medical therapy. Surgery should also be planned if there has been no improvement by around 5 days from the initiation of aggressive steroid therapy. Surgery is probably indicated in all patients in whom any monitoring criterion worsens, even if the overall status appears quite reasonable, and particularly so when the CRP level fails to fall or if one of the key radiological signs emerges. If in doubt, it is almost always safer to operate.

Table 1.1 Fulminant colitis: suggested framework for clinical and investigatory monitoring

Parameter	Frequency of monitoring
Pulse	6 hourly
Temperature	6 hourly
Stool frequency	Recorded on daily basis
Stool consistency	Recorded on daily basis
Presence of blood	Recorded on daily basis
Abdominal tenderness	Recorded on daily basis
Nature of bowel sounds	Recorded on daily basis
Serum electrolytes	Daily
Full blood count	Daily
Plain abdominal radiograph	Daily
Serum CRP	Thrice weekly
Serum albumin	Thrice weekly
'Global assessment'	Daily recorded as better, same or worse

There is probably only one operation to be considered in this context – subtotal colectomy with ileostomy formation (and probably a mucous fistula to vent the rectosigmoid colon). This aborts the emergency, avoids the danger of extensive pelvic dissection in the acute situation and permits elective pouch surgery to be considered at leisure. Even with this approach, colectomy for fulminant colitis has a mortality in the region of 5% (compared with less than 1% even for taxing, pouch-creating elective surgery).

A single episode of fulminant colitis – however catastrophic – once survived without surgery, curiously ceases to have any direct bearing on surgical planning for that patient. Although such patients do not escape future severe exacerbations, their risk of and their need for surgery are no greater (and may even be less) than those of other individuals with a similar disease extent.

Elective surgery

Surgery is rarely the first therapy considered in colitis, but it often proves an important component of the overall management of affected patients. In other than fulminant colitis, the decision will be an elective one with contributions to the decision-making process from physician, surgeon and patient, supported by ward and specialist nurses. When required, surgery is usually for uncontrolled chronic disease, with either a lack of adequate response to medical therapy, or steroid dependence. A careful analysis of the severity of symptoms and realistic expectations of surgery is essential in planning.

Surgery for ulcerative colitis should be almost synonymous with total colectomy because partial colectomy is usually followed by problematic relapse in the retained colon and because the patient is otherwise left at risk of colorectal carcinoma. Whether a total proctocolectomy with the formation of an end-ileostomy or a pouch reconstruction is then chosen is dealt with elsewhere in this volume.

Very occasionally, colectomy with ileorectal anastomosis will be considered in the young patient who is very keen to avoid an ileostomy but who is not ready to invest the time required for pouch creation. In this circumstance, a relatively generous portion of distal bowel should be left in continuity in order to avoid the need for two pelvic procedures.

Sexuality, fertility and pregnancy in ulcerative colitis

Great suffering can result from what may seem to be relatively minor defects in actual or perceived sexual functioning. Much has been written about the stigma of the gastrointestinal stoma, but less attention has been focused on the concern that faecal incontinence will occur during intercourse; this is much more often a worry than an actuality, but the anxiety of the patient (particularly the female sufferer) may be of such overwhelming intensity as to prevent the formation of any potentially sexual relationship.

It is typical of the whole area of sexual functioning that this major concern of patients is one which is not conveyed to their medical attendants: the doctor or nurse should recognize this and introduce its discussion at an appropriate point in the consulting process. Achieving secure continence may be difficult, but pre-coital loperamide may suffice and will often provide the reassurance that is needed. Dyspareunia is similarly a problem that is often not mentioned in the inflammatory bowel disease clinic, but it is about twice as common as in healthy women and should be enquired after in potentially sexually active women.

Males

In males, there are few problems apart from a temporarily reduced fertility when obviously sick, and reversible oligospermia from sulphasalazine. Alternative 5-ASA therapy should be chosen in a man planning a family. There are also hypothetical dangers to the fetus from the preconception exposure of the father to immunosuppressive drugs such as azathioprine.

Female fertility and pregnancy

The fertility of women with colitis is probably normal, although for reasons that are not clear the menopause occurs about 2 years earlier than in the general population.

Colitis typically runs a relatively benign course in pregnancy, around half of all women experiencing good-quality remission. There is a small proportion (10–15%) in whom the bowel is more troublesome, and colitis occasionally presents for the first time during pregnancy. It is common, however, for there to be relapse in the post-puerperal period.

Most of the drugs used in colitis are relatively innocuous in pregnancy. The 5-ASA drugs do not cross the placenta to any great extent, and there are no data indicating a risk to the fetus; thus, all of these can safely be used throughout pregnancy. Steroid use in pregnancy is emotive but unnecessarily so. There have been suggestions that cleft palate and hare-lip are more common in infants born to mothers on steroids, but the evidence for this is not compelling. With a daily systemic dose of less than 10 mg prednisolone (or 50 mg hydrocortisone), the risk of adrenal suppression in the infant is negligible, although adrenal problems can certainly affect the fetus and the neonate if larger doses are required for the mother's health. Alternatives to steroids should therefore be employed whenever possible, but the infant's health is best served by a full attention to its mother's needs.

None of the immunosuppressive agents should be used in pregnancy unless they are essential for maternal health, and methotrexate is always absolutely contraindicated. There are, however, reassuring data for azathioprine, which has been used without any discernible increase in fetal loss or abnormality.

Breast-feeding

Most drugs find their way into breast milk to some extent. Among those most likely to be used in colitis, there need be no greater anxiety than in pregnancy. Moderate doses of steroids given to the mother put the infant at risk of cosmetic changes and adrenal suppression (and possibly other steroid toxicity), but this is rarely a major issue. Breast-feeding is highly desirable but is not essential. If it is not possible for the mother to be satisfactorily maintained on a regime that is obviously safe for the infant, bottle-feeding is probably to be preferred.

Extra-intestinal manifestations

Joints

Ankylosing spondylitis and other spondarthritides are considerably more common in the colitic patient; these, however, run a course relatively independent from that of the colitis and need not be considered further.

There is also a condition peculiar to those with inflammatory bowel disease, the so-called inflammatory bowel disease-related arthropathy. This is common, affecting upwards of 15% of patients with colitis. It is usually a symmetrical polyarthropathy, affecting medium-sized joints. Radiological features are few, and a destructive arthritis does not occur. It follows an activity profile close but not identical to that of the associated colitis and tends to respond to gastrointestinal therapy (especially to steroids), but it may also have its onset or relapse as steroids are being withdrawn. Therapy is otherwise something of a problem since although non-steroidal anti-inflammatory agents are effective in many cases, they are often not tolerated because of a worsening of the colitis.

Osteoporosis

Bone density is undoubtedly reduced in patients with inflammatory bowel disease. This appears to reflect chronic disease activity at least as much as the use of steroids and is much more of a problem in Crohn's disease than in ulcerative colitis. Low bone density is never-theless found in many of patients with colitis. Fortunately, this amounts to osteoporosis in only 5–10% of cases.

Those involved in patient care should be aware of this, aim to mini-mize the use of steroids, encourage exercise and be alert to early intervention with hormone replacement therapy and bisphospho-nates if frank osteoporosis supervenes. Periodic bone density scans are now advised in all male colitics over the age of 50 and in post-menopausal women.

Skin problems

Erythema nodosum presents as painful, raised, red lesions, typically on the shins, at times of active colitis (Figure 1.6 and Plate 3). It affects about 2% of patients and usually runs a course parallel to that of the colitis without itself requiring therapy. It may recur with further exac-erbations of the colitis but very rarely recurs after proctocolectomy.

Pyoderma gangrenosum (Figure 1.7 and Plate 4) is a little less common; it is associated with long-standing disease, usually at times of active colitis. The lesions are typically single and on a lower limb.

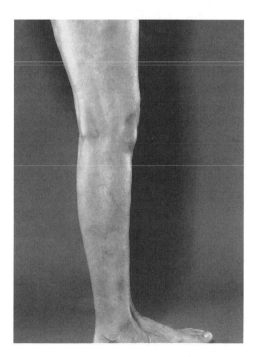

Figure 1.6: The multiple raised red lesions of erythema nodosum on the legs in patient with active ulcerative colitis (see Plate 3)

They develop into deep ulcers with a necrotic base, undermined purple edges and a purulent sterile discharge. Pyoderma gangrenosum may respond readily to colitis therapy, but, especially when there are many or large lesions, this is not the case, prolonged high-dose steroids, immunosuppression or even colectomy then possibly being indicated. Intralesional steroid injections and the application of potent steroid preparations beneath an impermeable dressing seem particularly helpful. Long-term scarring may remain.

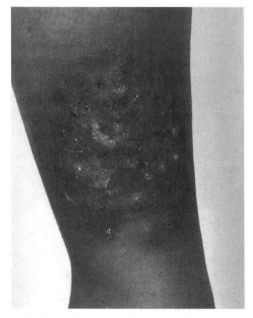

Figure 1.7 Characteristic appearances of pyoderma gangrenosum on the leg of a patient with active ulcerative colitis; note the colouration, the pus and the undermining of the ulcer edges; the beginnings of the cribiform scarring are also apparent (see Plate 4).

Ophthalmic complications

Iritis and uveitis present with a painful red eye and impaired visual acuity. The diagnosis can be confirmed by slit-lamp examination if it is not otherwise obvious. Topical steroids are usually sufficient therapy, but there is a risk of permanent damage if prompt treatment is not initiated.

Episcleritis is more common than uveitis and is usually responsible for redness and discomfort, with a conjunctivitis-like syndrome.

Treatment is not normally required, other than that for the concurrent active colitis, but topical steroids are occasionally needed.

Hepatobiliary disease in ulcerative colitis

The most important hepatobiliary disease associated with colitis is primary sclerosing cholangitis, but upwards of 10% of patients with ulcerative colitis have abnormal liver function tests at some time. In most cases these fortunately reflect active intestinal disease and have no other significance, but as well as sclerosing cholangitis, hepatic steatosis and certain forms of hepatitis are also over-represented.

Primary sclerosing cholangitis varies in both its severity and its tendency to progress. There is a characteristic pattern of inflammation and fibrosis, which causes a combination of stricturing and dilatation of the bile ducts within and outside the liver. Most patients (>80%) with primary sclerosing cholangitis also have ulcerative colitis, and about 2.5% of colitics develop primary sclerosing cholangitis. The colitis is usually both extensive and inactive.

Primary sclerosing cholangitis should be considered in all colitic patients who develop abnormal liver biochemistry. Early disease is almost always asymptomatic. With progression, cholestasis (pruritus, dark urine and pale stools), cholangitis and right upper quadrant abdominal pain start to occur. The diagnosis of primary sclerosing cholangitis currently requires endoscopic retrograde cholangiopancreatograpy (ERCP) and/or liver biopsy, but advances in magnetic resonance imaging may soon provide an adequate non-invasive alternative.

If a single dominant stricture is identified on ERCP, it is possible to dilate it with a transendoscopic balloon or splint it. Ursodeoxycholic acid may be of value in more diffuse disease, but end-stage liver disease responds only to liver transplantation. Female gender, increasing age, decreasing albumin level and increasing bilirubin are all poor prognostic markers. Patients with primary sclerosing cholangitis are also at a substantially increased risk of cholangiocarcinoma and of colorectal malignancy.

Thrombosis and thromboembolism in colitis

Deep vein thrombosis in the legs and pelvis, pulmonary embolism and mesenteric and intracranial thromboses are all over-represented in active colitis. A high level of abnormally sticky platelets and abnormalities of several serum factors contribute to this risk, exacerbated when the patient is immobile. This is beginning to take on medicolegal significance, and it will be difficult to refute future claims arising from thrombotic events if prophylactic measures have not been taken. All patients admitted for severe colitis should be on a prophylactic regime, preferably with subcutaneous heparin.

Malignancy complicating inflammatory bowel disease

Colorectal carcinoma is more common in those with long-standing extensive ulcerative colitis. The frequency of carcinoma is up to 5–10% at 20 years, rising to 12–30% at 30 years. There is little increase in risk in those with only left-sided disease, and a normal population risk in those with only proctitis.

Colonoscopic surveillance has therefore been practised. Published series indicate a (beneficial) higher frequency of Dukes' A and B tumours, and combining this with surgery for the premalignant dysplastic colon yields an overall cost for surveillance of around £30,000 for each life saved, which compares favourably with other surveillance programmes in the UK. Advanced cancers are still, however, encountered, and it is clear that surveillance strategies have so far been inadequate.

Taking up-to-date account of known and predicted influences, the following is currently advocated. All patients with colitis should have a colonoscopy at 8–10 years unless the upper limit of disease has always been seen on prior sigmoidoscopy. If macroscopic extensive disease (at any time proximal to the splenic flexure) is documented, surveillance should commence. Surveillance is also legitimate if there is macroscopic left-sided disease, as well as if there is one first-order relative with colorectal carcinoma, or a personal history of colorectal adenoma or primary sclerosing cholangitis, but not if there is only microscopic disease.

Surveillance may sensibly comprise full colonoscopy every 2 years with at least 10 biopsies at no more than 10 cm intervals, and flexible sigmoidoscopy (or colonoscopy) with multiple biopsies in the intervening years. If high-grade dysplasia or cancer develops, surgery is essential. If there is confirmed low-grade dysplasia (two sites or two occasions with two pathologists), surgery is strongly advised.

CHAPTER 2

Familial adenomatous polyposis

KAY NEALE AND ROBIN PHILLIPS

Colorectal cancer is the second most common cancer in non-smoking men and women. Althoug lung cancer is in numerical terms more common, it is usually caused by smoking. Breast cancer is also more common in women, but since men rarely develop it, colorectal cancer is overall more significant.

Colorectal cancer arises from a particular type of polyp, the adenoma. It can arise in flat mucosa, particularly in long-standing ulcerative colitis, through a dysplasia–carcinoma sequence and, much more importantly, via an adenoma–carcinoma sequence. Few patients have a strong family history of colorectal cancer, but in those who do, there is often a genetic element. In some people, this genetic element may be relatively weak and give rise to a tendency towards colorectal cancer, but in others it may be so strong as to be considered dominantly inherited.

The two most important dominantly inherited colorectal cancer syndromes are hereditary non-polyposis colorectal cancer (HNPCC) and familial adenomatous polyposis (FAP). In HNPCC, there may well be a history of other cancers, particularly gynaecological, and polyps in the bowel are absent or scarce. In this chapter, however, we are concerned with FAP, in which many hundreds or even thousands of colorectal adenomas may be seen.

Historical background to FAP

FAP is a rare, genetically inherited disease that affects the whole body. Diagnosis has traditionally depended on the presence of more than one hundred adenomatous polyps in the colon and rectum. Nowadays, it is often possible to identify the genetic mutation responsible and offer diagnosis before the polyps appear or in patients in whom the number of polyps visible to the naked eye is less than one hundred (Figure 2.1).

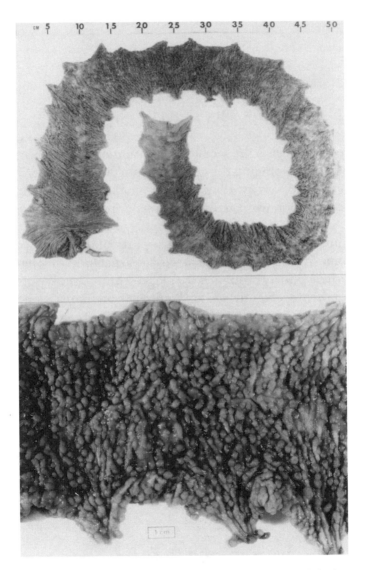

Figure 2.1 Transection of the colon with many polyps, hence familial adenomatous polyposis.

FAP is an autosomal dominant condition caused by a mutation of the APC gene, which lies on the long arm of chromosome 5. The gene is huge, classically consisting of 15 coding parts known as exons, the areas of DNA between them being known as introns. The gene codes for a protein that seems to be important in cell-to-cell adhesion. Mutations of the gene are important in sporadic colorectal cancer as well as in FAP. The reason why such a condition affecting the whole body is classed as a colorectal disease is that the average age of death, from colorectal cancer, in people carrying the faulty gene is 39 years unless they receive surgical treatment.

The study of FAP at St Mark's Hospital was started by Dr Cuthbert Dukes in 1924, long before prophylactic surgical treatment was readily available. Major surgery of the type undertaken today would usually have resulted in the death of the patient from infection or shock as antibiotics were not available and electrolyte balance was not understood. The doctors who recognized the condition in these early years often discovered that the patient had a family history of early death from cancer, but all they could do for their own patient was wait for a malignancy to occur and remove it, and then wait for the next.

During this time, a register was kept at St Mark's of these families. The register included detailed information that enabled Dr Dukes, some 20 years after the start of the polyposis register, to explain that polyposis was inherited in a Mendelian dominant manner and could be transmitted by either parent to children of both sexes. This means that every child born to a parent with FAP has a 50 per cent chance of inheriting it.

On 8th December 1948, the first colectomy with ileorectal anastomosis (IRA) for FAP at St Mark's Hospital was carried out by Mr O. V. Lloyd Davies. Around this period, some surgeons felt that it was dangerous to leave the rectum intact, and over the years that followed, the main thrust of research in the Polyposis Registry was to determine the long-term results of the IRA.

At this time, it was, however, recognized that a form of treatment avoiding a stoma, and therefore acceptable to patients, was available. It was now sensible actively to record the family history, with the aim of identifying the people who were at risk of inheriting the condition in order to offer them screening and treatment.

Knudson's hypothesis

Why do inherited cancer cases tend to develop often multiple cancers at a young age? The present explanation is known as Knudson's hypothesis, and it involves the following. Everyone will inherit one of each pair of chromosomes from their mother and one from their father. These chromosomes will contain genes, either maternally or paternally derived, which are known as alleles. Knudson supposed that both alleles of a recessive gene had to be knocked out or faulty in some way for cancer to develop.

In sporadic cases of cancer, both 'hits' have to occur via environmental means. This unlikely combination of events clearly happens infrequently and occurs only over a prolonged period of time. Hence sporadic tumours tend to be single and occur in the elderly. If, however, one 'hit' has been inherited in the germ line, it only takes one other hit on the other allele anywhere in the vast colonic mucosal surface for an adenoma to be initiated – the first step on the path to cancer. This is obviously much more likely than the first scenario, which is why multiple polyps (and hence multiple cancers) tend to develop at a young age in these patients.

Screening

Over the years since the IRA was first developed, various screening programmes have been initiated. The advice given to patients at St Mark's is constantly under review, modifications being made in the light of new experience. Until recently, the only way to tell whether a person had inherited FAP from a parent was to look into the bowel to see whether any polyps had developed. If none was seen, the patient would be told that all was clear at that moment but that he or she must return for another examination the same time the following year.

It had long been agreed that the age at which asymptomatic children should be encouraged to be examined was 14. Children younger than this complaining of symptoms needed examination and advice, but it was considered important that, in the absence of symptoms, they should not delay much beyond their fourteenth birthday. The reasoning behind this was that the condition was in some cases sufficiently advanced by this age that surgical treatment needed to be planned immediately. The other reason was that parents could usually persuade children of that age to attend hospital for examination. Once they were older, the children sometimes refused screening, with disastrous results. It should be noted that colorectal cancer has been seen in patients with FAP as young as 17 years of age.

The age at which a patient can be safely discharged from a screening programme is constantly debated. At St Mark's, patients are rarely formally discharged, but the screening interval is lengthened as age increases into the fourth and fifth decades. There are some families in which the polyps always seem to develop early and some in which they always seem to develop late. But just when it looks as though a pattern can be predicted, someone from a family in which polyps develop early will, after years of clear screening examinations, turn up for their annual review and be found to be affected.

Finally, after years of research, the gene causing FAP was localized to the long arm of chromosome 5 (Bodmer et al 1987), and in 1991, the exact position of the gene was discovered. It was, however, another 5 years before an NHS diagnostic DNA service for FAP families was set up by St Mark's at the Kennedy Galton Centre, Northwick Park.

Even now, things are not completely straightforward. The genetic mutation, that is the change (or fault) in the gene, differs from family to family. This means that DNA from an affected person in a family must be available for use by the molecular geneticists in order to identify the particular mutation running in that family. Only then can those at risk of inheriting the condition have a blood test to determine whether they have the faulty gene or the normal gene. Even when DNA is available, the test is so complex that, using the methods currently available, the abnormality in the gene can only be identified in 60–70 per cent of families.

Mutation testing

Imagine the APC gene as a long train consisting of 15 carriages. Somewhere, anywhere, on that train there is a fault. It could be electrical, mechanical, anything. To find that fault would require the whole train to be taken apart, carriage by carriage, and at the end of it all, if the fault is minor, it may even pass unnoticed. This is the situation that occurs when the laboratory sets out to isolate an unknown mutation in a polyposis family.

As FAP is clinically obvious (because it has an obvious phenotype), it is worthwhile undertaking this laborious task in a confirmed case. Many patients, however, simply do not know for sure whether their relative actually had polyposis or just polyps. What makes matters worse, many pathologists do not make the difference clear in their histopathology reports.

It is here that a Polyposis Registry can be of assistance. The original histological blocks can be traced so that they can be reviewed by a pathologist knowledgeable in intestinal disorders in general and polyposis in particular. If the case is confirmed as one of FAP, detecting mutations in a DNA sample from a known affected individual is worthwhile. It is not worthwhile, however, performing mutation analysis just on the offchance. There is no point going through the hugely laborious process of taking the APC gene apart, block by block, if there is even a reasonable chance that there may be nothing (inherited) wrong with it in the first place.

Let us now consider a polyposis family in whom the mutation has been detected. It is then a fairly simple matter to look for that mutation in at-risk family members. Returning to the analogy of the train, if a bolt is missing from under the back seat, on the left, in the fifteenth carriage, it is easy to send an engineer in to check other trains for a similar problem. Indeed, this is exactly what is done when a fault is found in a new car and all similar cars are recalled for a check.

In practice, mutation testing is still in its infancy. It may not be available, or the mutation in a family may not be known. Thus, clinical screening is still the mainstay of the management of at-risk individuals. Such individuals are usually seen clinically for the first time in their early teenage years. Parents are encouraged to bring younger children with them when they themselves visit in order for them to become comfortable and familiar with regular attendance at hospital, but these children will not be examined.

From the age of 14 years, annual rigid sigmoidoscopy is commenced, looking for polyps in the rectum. When polyps are present, it is usual for one or two to be visible in the rectum, but they can be overlooked, and there may even be rectal sparing. For this reason, colonoscopy is usually advised, being performed first at the age of 20 and 5 yearly thereafter. Colonoscopy is not advocated earlier because cancer is unusual in youngsters with polyposis, and on the rare occasion that it does occur, the polyposis tends to be dense and easily recognizable on rigid sigmoidoscopy.

It is important to remember, when dealing with polyposis patients, that, in the absence of a genetic test, lifelong surveillance will be necessary. If gentleness and tact are lacking, the patient may very well decide not to re-attend. What is worse, he or she may persuade other at-risk family members not to be screened either. It therefore usually pays for experienced health-care professionals to see these patients, and it is often more important to perform some form of sigmoidoscopy comfortably and discreetly rather than the most thorough examination with indignity and discomfort; there will always be another opportunity next year. It is important too to keep an accurate and up-to-date family tree to identify new family members. Registry staff are invaluable in this respect.

Patients presenting for the first time with polyposis are usually older and symptomatic. New mutations account for about 20 per cent of polyposis cases, and these patients will of course lack a family history. It is nevertheless important to screen their parents and any siblings once just to be sure. In these cases, full colonoscopy employing a technique called dye spray is called for. Again, Registry staff will help to track down all such family members and offer them screening.

Treatment

The treatment of affected polyposis patients is surgical, but there are those who have argued for screening with or without chemoprevention. Various non-steroidal anti-inflammatory drugs (and newer derivatives) will cause polyp regression. This is, however, frequently incomplete, and cancer has been reported to have developed in patients while they are on treatment. Furthermore, screening is neither 100 per cent accurate nor 100 per cent safe. Why switch a, probably inevitable, operation for cancer prevention for a later operation trying harder for cancer cure?

The first essential is to remove or minimize the risk of colorectal cancer. Polyposis patients are prone to a range of other problems, such as polyps in the upper gastrointestinal tract, desmoid tumours and thyroid cancer. The importance of these is, however, minor compared with the importance of their large bowel disease.

Surgical options

The surgical choices are:

- colectomy with IRA;
- restorative proctocolectomy with the construction of an ileo-anal pouch (RPC);
- proctocolectomy with permanent end-ileostomy.

A proctocolectomy and permanent end-ileostomy should really now only ever be considered in the presence of a low rectal cancer. In this day and age, patients advised to have this operation should be counselled to seek a second opinion in order to be sure that it really is necessary and that they have indeed given their full consent to it.

Surgeons debate endlessly between the choices of the colectomy with IRA or RPC (the pouch procedure). The rationale for each is described below.

IRA

A colectomy with IRA is a simple, low-morbidity operation with a good functional result. It is suitable for the young because their rectal cancer risk is extremely low and because the anticipated lack of complications means that they are unlikely to experience severe disruption to their schooling. It is probably not suited for those who have dense polyposis, even if they are young, whereas it might be considered in older patients with a more attenuated, low-density form of polyposis.

Lifelong 6 monthly examination of the rectal stump will be necessary to check for dense rectal polyposis, large adenomas or cancer. The risk of rectal cancer after IRA is 8 per cent by 50 years old but rises to 30 per cent by the age of 60. Most patients found to have rectal cancer will, however, be cured of it surgically. Consideration should be given to the removal of the rectum with the construction of an ileo-anal pouch if the rectal polyps become uncontrollable, or as patients become older.

Ileo-anal pouch

A proctocolectomy with the construction of an ileo-anal pouch is a more complex operation, with a significantly higher in-hospital complication rate. In the few cases in whom the operation is a failure, a permanent ileostomy may become necessary. A temporary ileostomy is frequently advised to assist the pouch to heal.

The operation does remove the risk of subsequent rectal cancer, but as upper gastrointestinal cancer is the leading cause of death after IRA, rectal cancer is not the only consideration. The pouches themselves are prone to subsequent polyp development and have an unknown, albeit probably very small, cancer risk. Thus, rectal cancer risk should not weigh the decision too heavily against the alternative of an IRA.

On the whole, the ileo-anal pouch is probably best suited to those patients with dense polyposis irrespective of age, and to older patients because the risk of rectal cancer closer to the age of 50 is considerably greater. Both the surgical options described here will be discussed in greater detail within this book.

Associated conditions

Non-life-threatening extra-colonic manifestations of FAP

In addition to colorectal polyps, there are other manifestations of FAP that may alert the doctor to the diagnosis. These include the presence of lumps or bumps on the body, which may be either sebaceous cysts or osteomas. Patients with FAP may also report a history of having had dental abnormalities such as funny or extra teeth. Epidermoid cysts are benign, soft, subcutaneous tumours, which may appear anywhere on the body. It is not necessary to remove these cysts unless they are unsightly or inconveniently placed. Osteomas most commonly develop in the cranium and mandibles; also benign, they tend to show local growth.

Some patients with polyposis may have pigmentation on the retina, which is known as congenital hypertrophy of the retinal pigment epithelium, or CHRPE (pronounced 'chirpy'). As some normal individuals occasionally have similar (albeit not identical) pigmentation, and not all patients with FAP have CHRPE, fundoscopy is not very useful clinically.

The upper gastrointestinal tract

Almost all polyposis patients can be shown to have duodenal adenomas, and about half have gastric fundic polyps. However, whereas with the large bowel component of polyposis, the risk of cancer if left untreated is virtually 100 per cent, with the duodenum the risk of cancer is about 5 per cent. The gastric fundic gland polyps, although they can appear pretty impressive at endoscopy, are probably not relevant in cancer risk terms. Apart from in Japan, there is little or no increased risk of gastric cancer in polyposis patients despite half of them having these polyps.

Nobody really knows how to manage duodenal polyposis. Various trials of different treatments are underway, and it is hoped that some form of chemopreventative agent will ultimately be successfully developed. Duodenal polyposis is staged by the Spigelman classification, stages I and II being mild and III and IV severe disease. It is currently recommended that upper gastrointestinal screening with a side-viewing video-duodenoscope commences at around 25 years of age. In Spigelman stages I and II, the screening interval might thereafter be 5 years, but with stage III and IV disease more frequent examinations are called for. In the worst cases, 6 monthly screening and sometimes prophylactic pylorus-preserving duodenectomy may be necessary.

Desmoid disease

Desmoid tumours are fibromatous masses of tissue, conceptually rather like huge uterine fibroids although, histologically and behaviourally, entirely different (Figure 2.2). Although they may occur sporadically in patients who do not have FAP, the diagnosis of a desmoid tumour should nevertheless alert the clinician to the possibility of FAP.

These tumours are locally invasive but do not metastasize. They occur in about 10 per cent of polyposis cases and are an important cause of death in treated patients. The average survival of polyposis patients treated by colectomy and IRA is extended by 30 years compared with historical, untreated controls. Nevertheless, this

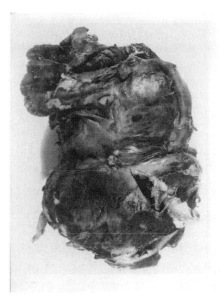

Figure 2.2 Desmoid tumour.

survival still falls 10 years short of that of the general population, desmoid disease being an important reason for this.

Desmoid tumours can be classified as body wall or intra-abdominal. Body wall desmoids can be successfully excised with a reasonably good chance of cure, although extensive defects may need subsequent plastic surgical repair. Intra-abdominal desmoids are, however, quite another matter. They infiltrate the mesentery of the small intestine and encroach on the superior mesenteric artery. In the retroperitoneum, they can compress the ureters, leading to hydronephrosis and renal failure. Surgical removal is hazardous and is usually only attempted in desperate cases.

It is common for desmoid tissue to adhere to other structures, making it impossible to remove the whole tumour, which leads to early recurrence. It is also felt that the surgical trauma may itself cause the desmoid disease to grow more aggressively. Where the desmoid is adhered to other structures, it may be impossible to remove that particular structure. If a large length of small bowel is removed, the patient may become reliant upon intravenous nutrition. Desmoid tumours also tend to be very vascular, giving a significant risk of intra-operative haemorrhage. Encapsulated tumours have, however, been successfully removed (Berk et al 1992).

Alternative treatments include the non-steroidal anti-inflammatory drug sulindac, tamoxifen or its alternative toremifene and, in particularly aggressive cases, cytotoxic chemotherapy with doxorubicin and dacarbazine (Figure 2.3).

Other problems

Polyposis patients are also at risk of a variety of other benign and malignant neoplasms, from adrenal adenomas through to other cancers, particularly of the thyroid. Nevertheless, the majority of treated polyposis patients can still expect a reasonable life expectancy with good quality of life.

Survival

As stated above, the average survival of polyposis patients treated by colectomy with IRA is extended by 30 years compared with

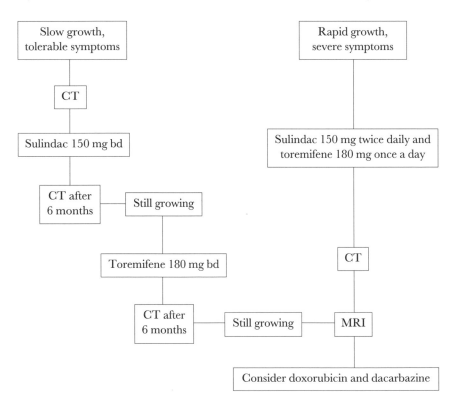

Figure 2.3 Treatment recommendation for intra-abdominal desmoids.

historical, untreated controls. The 10 year shortfall in survival compared with that of the general population is largely due to desmoid disease and upper gastrointestinal malignancy.

The Polyposis Registry

The management of polyposis patients is hugely facilitated by Registries, of which there are a number within the UK. The London area is served by the St Mark's Hospital Polyposis Registry, founded in 1924 and the oldest and largest in the world, and Regional Genetic Centres.

FAP or not?

Two types of new patient may be referred to hospital because of polyposis: those who are said to have polyposis and those who are said to have a relative with polyposis. If the new patient is said to have polyposis and still has their colon, there is usually no difficulty in determining the exact diagnosis. The colon can be examined, the polyps counted and biopsies taken to confirm that they are adenomas.

   If the patient has already had the colon and rectum removed, or if he or she has been referred for screening because a parent is said to have had FAP, the Registry will contact the hospital where the surgery was carried out. Pathology reports or pathological slides will be obtained so that a specialist colorectal pathologist can confirm the diagnosis. It is essential not to confuse FAP with other types of polyposis, or with any another type of hereditary bowel cancer, because the screening programme for those at risk is quite different.

Tracing and tracking

At St Mark's Hospital, the work in the Polyposis Registry has changed considerably over the years. It was the pathologist Dr Cuthbert Dukes who first had the idea of starting a register of polyposis patients. He was a Quaker, a very humane man with an overriding desire to ensure that his work, and the research carried out at St Mark's, led to an improvement in the quality of people's lives. In 1958, he stated, 'it would be difficult to find a more promising field for the exercise of cancer control than a polyposis family because both diagnosis and treatment are possible in the precancerous stage and because the results of surgical treatment are excellent' (Dukes 1958).

We can see today that this is quite clearly true. Registry statistics show that if patients who have the polyposis gene wait until they have symptoms before requesting medical advice, 66 per cent will already have a colorectal malignancy. Of the relatives who are traced and informed of their risk, and who agree to undergo screening, only 5 per cent have colorectal malignancy when seen. But taking family details from one relative and telling that person to warn the other family members that they should see their doctor is not enough.

The exercise of taking a complete and detailed family history is time consuming and may be laborious. It is, of course, never completed because the structure of a family changes with time, but in addition to that there are often secrets, details that are only divulged once the giver is satisfied that the receiver of those details both is to be trusted and will not be critical. Family pedigrees are thus built up over time. Making contact with the relatives who are identified as being 'at risk' is also a lengthy process.

Most relatives are eager to learn about the condition and to do everything they can to be screened and to encourage their brothers, sisters and children to be screened, but some are very reluctant. A whole variety of reasons are given for not wanting, or not being able, to visit the hospital. These include such things as 'I can't take time from work', 'It didn't do my mother/father much good', 'I believe in the healing power of prayer' or 'My GP says that if I feel all right, I don't need to come'.

The Registry staff need to be able to talk through such issues and assess how much pressure to apply. In some cases, it may take years to persuade someone to agree to a screening test. It is important to have in place a system that enables reluctant people to be monitored over a long period of time because too much pressure all at once may result in an outright refusal and an order not to bother them again. It is much better to be less pushy, to be alert and sympathetic to their difficulties, and in the longer term to be successful in persuading them to attend.

Registry staff monitor the attendance of patients at St Mark's Hospital either for follow-up after surgery or for screening examinations prior to diagnosis. They also contact people who do not turn up for an outpatient appointment to find out why and arrange a new appointment at a convenient time. When several appointments have been missed and contacting a patient proves difficult, staff write to the GP to alert him or her to the situation. The care received by those patients attending St Mark's is multidisciplinary. Various disciplines are needed to cope with the burden placed upon a family living with polyposis, which is quite considerable. There are, of course, the psychological stresses and strains arising from, for example, fear, guilt and blame, as well as the rarer life-threatening complications of the disease.

Leaving this aside, the number of hospital visits required each year simply to keep the disease under review can be difficult for a working adult or a mother with young children. If the patient has a minor problem, such as a large polyp that needs to be removed, or a bout of obstructive symptoms caused by adhesions, more visits and perhaps a night or two as an inpatient add to the time away from work or to problems with childcare. If a child or another relative is admitted, more journeys to the hospital as a visitor are undertaken. By playing a role in coordinating these visits, the Registry staff can minimize the amount of travelling and the time lost from work. For those patients who find coping particularly difficult and for those trying to deal with rarer complications, referral to the medical social worker can be arranged. Similarly, emergency appointments can be easily arranged by a telehone call to the Registry.

Research

Polyposis patients generously give their time to help in research, but clinicians should be sympathetic to the many requests they receive and be wary of overburdening them. By using the Polyposis Registry database, Registry staff are able to identify patients who meet study criteria, and by using their personal knowledge of the families, they can advise researchers which patients should not be approached because of unhappy or difficult personal circumstances.

Because of the hereditary nature of polyposis, sufferers are usually very keen to take part in research, many feeling guilty if they refuse. Knowing this, it would be unfair for us to burden them by taking advantage of their feelings; indeed, if we did so, they would probably respond by failing to turn up for their appointments. Thus, by getting to know the individuals and by working with them to make their lives as normal as possible, we are able to keep a cohort of willing subjects.

By continuing to come to St Mark's for care, each patient plays a part in helping us to learn more about polyposis and how it should be treated. Regardless of whether or not patients take part in specific studies, their progress is recorded at the Registry. In this way, we constantly review such things as which type of surgery gives the best outcome, whether the screening programme is effective and what associated conditions are causing patients most problems. It is this general, ongoing research that often leads the way to a change of policy or to a more intense, specific research project.

Helpline

The Polyposis Registry staff are available to talk to anyone about polyposis and can be contacted during normal working hours (see Useful Addresses). If they cannot answer questions immediately, advice can usually be given on where the required information can be found.

CHAPTER 3

Carcinoma of the rectum

JOHN NORTHOVER, CLAIRE TAYLOR AND DARREN GOLD

Cancer of the rectum is very common; in Western countries, counted in both men and women, and combined with colonic cancer, it lies second in the league table of malignant causes of death. Among non-smoking males, who are the clear majority, colon and rectal cancers are the most common cancer killers.

In the UK, there are around 30,000 new cases annually, of whom nearly 20,000 are destined to die of the disease, split roughly equally between rectum and colon. In many Western countries, the condition is even more common, while in many urbanizing countries, as in the UK during the nineteenth century, it is climbing in incidence and hence importance as a public health issue. Globally, colorectal cancer is the fourth most common cancer killer, with 875,000 cases annually, accounting for 8.5 per cent of all new cases (Potter 1996); in 1996, there were 510,000 colorectal cancer deaths worldwide, 7.2 per cent of all cancer deaths.

This chapter discusses the various aspects of rectal cancer – why it occurs, who it affects, how it is treated and how it might be prevented – there are some areas in which it is so inextricably part of bowel cancer (i.e. including colonic cancer) that those sections will address the wider field. Other areas, such as the surgery of the disease, will consider rectal cancer alone.

Demographic details

Geography

Bowel cancer is predominantly a disease of 'developed' countries, having been a major cause of cancer death in Europe, North America

43

and the UK's former Dominions for much of the twentieth century. As countries or subsections of national populations become more affluent, and perhaps because of their adoption of 'Western' habits and diets, they begin to take on the higher bowel cancer risks of the West.

There is an enormous variation in the incidence of colorectal cancer between countries: up to a 200-fold variation in rectal cancer incidence in men. Japanese men in Hawaii, the descendants of migrants, are twice as likely to develop rectal cancer as their cousins in Japan. These classic observations were part of the evidence that environmental factors, particularly diet, play a major role in the aetiology of colorectal cancer. The widest male–female difference is seen in Hawaiian Polynesians (28 and 14 per 100,000 respectively) (Parkin et al 1987).

Age

Bowel cancer is predominantly a disease of late middle and old age. The median age for this condition is 70 years, only 3 per cent of cases occurring before the age of 45 years.

Gender

The most comprehensive data on gender difference in colorectal cancer incidence and mortality are available from the USA. These data, derived for the Surveillance, Epidemiology and End Results (SEER) programme, indicate that there is a significant difference in age-adjusted colorectal cancer mortality between males and females, and that blacks are more frequently affected than whites.

Changes in incidence and mortality by gender and time

SEER data indicate that the incidence of colorectal cancer increased in males in the period 1950–84, whilst it fell slightly in females. From the mid-1980s onwards, there has been a steady decline in incidence in both sexes (Chu et al 1994).

Pathogenesis

There is no evidence that the factors that lead to rectal cancer are any different from those causing colonic cancer, so the two should be examined together. Our understanding of the pathogenesis of colorectal cancer developed first in conventional pathological terms and then, over the past 10 years, at the molecular level.

Unlike the other common cancers, colorectal cancer usually passes through an orderly pathological sequence, known as the adenoma–carcinoma sequence (ACS), in which normal mucosa becomes dysplastic and then develops small benign adenomas that usually become raised, making them visible macroscopically (Muto et al 1975). A proportion of these go on to become larger adenomas, and some may ultimately undergo malignant change, utlimately metastasizing to lymph nodes and distant sites (Gutman & Fidler 1995). Probably fewer than 1 per cent of adenomas progress to malignancy (Hamilton 1996), the malignant tissue soon overgrowing and destroying the adenoma (Figure 3.1).

Much more recently, a series of genetic alterations – mostly occurring in tissues exposed to the causative environmental factors, although some can be inherited mutations – have been identified that are causally related to the macroscopic elements of the ACS (Fearson & Vogelstein 1990). In a small proportion of individuals, perhaps around 5 per cent, dominantly inherited mutations induce a very high risk of colorectal cancer at an early age.

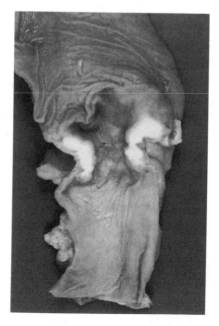

Figure 3.1 Adenocarcinoma of the rectum (see Plate 5).

Causative factors

As the incidence rate of this condition varies 20-fold around the world, it is highly likely that environmental – mainly dietary – factors play a major part in the aetiology of this condition. Certain epidemiological associations are consistently, and strongly, seen: high levels of dietary meat protein and fat, and a low intake of vegetables, appear to play a major part. Hereditary predisposition plays a much smaller role in the general population.

Lifestyle and environmental factors

Diet

The most consistent dietary observation is that vegetable consumption is inversely proportional to bowel cancer risk (Potter et al 1993). A high fibre intake appears similarly protective, although cereal intake seems to be proportionately related to cancer risk in Italy and Japan (Potter 1996). Data on the protective effects of fruit are more limited and inconsistent (Potter 1996).

The consumption of animal protein is generally associated with bowel cancer risk, although fish and seafood may show an inverse relationship (Potter et al 1993). The specific mechanisms whereby animal fat predisposes to bowel cancer are unclear, the presence of fat and the processing and cooking methods being possible factors (Potter 1996). Heavily browned meat, with a consequent excess of mutagenic heterocyclic amines, may be an important meat-related factor (Gerhardsson-de-Verdier et al 1991).

Evidence concerning calcium and vitamin D intake has been conflicting. Although the intake of various micronutrients, such as selenium and the carotenoids, has been said to be protective, the quality of the evidence and the inferences that can be drawn from individual studies leaves this complex area far from clear and certainly without sufficient support to warrant the dietary advice that has been given (Potter 1996).

Physical activity

It has become apparent in both sexes that physical inactivity is associated with increasing colon cancer risk (Slattery et al 1990). The lifetime pattern is probably more important than the effect of a relatively recent change in lifestyle; the association with rectal cancer has been less often examined and is less apparent.

Occupation

Besides their relevance in relation to physical activity, some occupations may expose workers to specific substances carrying risk; asbestos, with a doubling of bowel cancer risk excess is the best documented, although pesticide and herbicide exposure may also carry some risk. Painters, printers, railwaymen and wood and car workers have all been shown to be more highly affected (Potter 1996).

Smoking

Although cigarette smoking has not been implicated, cigar and pipe smoking have, in case control studies, been shown to be more common (Potter 1996).

Alcohol

A bare majority of 19 population studies have shown a positive correlation between bowel cancer risk and alcohol intake (Potter 1996). Beer consumption appears to be more positively correlated with rectal cancer in men than in women. It is likely that the association is related to the total ethanol intake rather then the type of drink consumed.

Caffeine

The few studies in this area have produced conflicting data. Overall, evidence suggests that coffee may decrease colorectal cancer risk (Potter 1996).

Heredity

This is a small factor in terms of overall effect (see the section on high-risk groups below).

Clinical features

Symptoms

Rectal cancer often presents with symptoms at a late stage in the evolution of the disease: in some series as many as 50 per cent of cases are manifestly beyond cure by the time that symptoms compel sufferers to seek help. This is caused partly by the sometimes advanced stage of the disease before it produces symptoms, and partly by the delay in presentation after symptom onset. The symptoms of rectal cancer may be mistaken for those of more minor conditions such as haemorrhoids or irritable bowel syndrome by the patient, the general practitioner or both, leading to further delay (Holliday & Hardcastle 1979, Crosland & Jones 1995). The most common symptoms are:

- *A change in bowel habit.* This may be a minor change in the frequency or timing of defaecation, or an unexplained change in stool consistency. Moreover, there is often a variation and irregularity in the frequency and consistency of the stool. This symptom was, in a recent case control study, shown to be the best diagnostic discriminator (Curless et al 1994)
- *Bleeding.* Blood may be seen to be mixed with the motion. Various shades of colour of the blood may be seen: it is usually bright red in rectal cancer, although no shade is site specific. In people at and beyond middle age, rectal bleeding has a positive predictive value for cancer of at least 10% (Goulston & Dent 1986, Fitjen et al 1995).
- *Mucous discharge.* This may be prominent, often stained by stool or blood.
- *Tenesmus.* A rectal tumour can give a sensation of incomplete evacuation as 'malignant stool' remains firmly attached to the rectal wall.
- *Symptoms of acute complications.* Around 30 per cent of all bowel tumours present as emergencies with obstruction or peritonitis (Goulston 1980, Chester & Britton 1989), although rectal cancers rarely present this way.

Any of these symptoms should lead the patient, particularly if middle aged or elderly, to seek medical advice.

Signs

General signs of anaemia and/or weight loss should be sought. Abdominal examination may reveal that the liver is enlarged as a result of metastasis.

Digital examination should always be a part of the examination of the patient presenting with any of the above symptoms. A rectal tumour up to 10 cm from the anus may be palpable as a firm, sometimes ulcerated mass arising from the rectal wall. Even if the tumour is not palpable, blood or mucous on the glove may provide a clue. Rigid sigmoidoscopy is a routine part of outpatient examination, permitting the distal 25 cm of colon and rectum to be examined.

Investigation of the suspected case

In the patient suspected of suffering from rectal cancer, investigation aims to confirm the diagnosis, establish the local extent of the tumour and look for evidence of distant spread. The two major methods of investigation in cases of suspected bowel cancer are endoscopy and radiology.

Endoscopy

Colonoscopy has become more widely used as the investigation of choice; it allows the biopsy of any identified lesion and is more sensitive than contrast radiology in the detection of small cancers and adenomas. A small proportion of cancers are identified as malignant polyps on endoscopy and may be treated definitively by endoscopic polypectomy. Colonoscopy should be performed to check the rest of the large bowel as around 5 per cent of patients will be found to have a second cancer; upstream adenomas need to be identified and removed to prevent their possible progression to malignancy. It must be remembered that colonoscopy carries a small but definite morbidity and mortality (Winawer et al 1997).

Radiology

In the process of confirming the presence of a rectal primary tumour, radiology has little part to play. A double-contrast barium enema may be used as an alternative to colonoscopy to examine the rest of the large bowel. Its shortcomings in relation to endoscopy are mentioned above.

Preoperative staging

As treatment planning becomes more complex, preoperative staging investigations to define the anatomy of the primary tumour and any locoregional or distant spread become more important. This process facilitates decisions not only about the nature of the surgery, but also about the various possible preoperative adjuvant therapies.

The primary tumour can be scanned using whole-body methods such as computed tomography (CT) or magnetic resonance imaging (MRI), or more localized procedures, for example liver ultrasound (US) and intrarectal US or MRI (Malone & McGrath 1993). Using intrarectal US, a well-established technique, rectal tumours can be reliably examined to provide evidence regarding the degree of spread through the rectal wall and the possible involvement of contiguous organs (Hildebrandt & Feifel 1995).

Management of rectal cancer

Surgery

In 1908, Ernest Miles described his radical operation for rectal cancer, based on the tenets of radical surgery defined by Halstad some years earlier. There was now, for the first time, an operation that offered the chance of cure for this increasingly prevalent condition (Miles 1908). Miles' operation was controversial because of its high operative death rate – around 40 per cent – but for the next 30 years, any rectal cancer patient in whom cure was to be attempted was likely to be offered Miles' abdominoperineal excision and permanent colostomy.

By 1940, as a result of the work of pathologists such as Cuthbert Dukes from St Mark's Hospital, the lymphatic drainage of the rectum was sufficiently well understood (predominantly in a cephalad direction, away from the anus) for it to be suggested that, in upper, and later in mid, rectal cancers, sphincter-saving surgery could be offered without compromising the chance of cure (Dukes 1929, Dixon 1939).

The rest of the twentieth century saw improvements in techniques and technology that have allowed the proportion of sphincter-saving operations to increase, so that today around 75 per cent of potentially curable cases can expect such surgery in specialist centres (Parks 1972, Williams et al 1985, Heald & Ryall 1986).

Internationally, a major issue in rectal cancer surgical technique has been the radicality of surgery; most Japanese surgeons have opted for procedures that incorporate an extended lymphadectomy, involving the wide excision of lymph nodes on the posterior abdominal and pelvic side walls (Hojo et al 1989). This technique, which the Japanese hold to be more generally curative, has the considerable disadvantage of regular and considerable damage to the autonomic innervation of the pelvis, manifesting as interference with bladder sensation and emptying, as well as impotence in males.

In the UK and the rest of Europe, a re-emphasis on the importance of the complete circumferential clearance of the mesorectum, rather than extending the operation in the manner of Japanese surgeons, has led to a clearer view of the nature of 'good' rectal cancer surgery (Quirke et al 1986, Heald & Karanjia 1992).

Over the past 40 years, the evolution in surgical technique has been seen as offering less mutilating surgery while maintaining rather than improving the cure rate of rectal cancer; surgery was, to a major extent, taken for granted as the basis of treatment, while the hunt for improvements in prognosis has centred on adjuvant therapy. In the past decade, however, surgeons have sought evidence of a variation in outcome related directly to the surgeon who is operating, and therefore for elements of the surgical procedure that might affect prognosis (Phillips et al 1983, McArdle & Hole 1991).

It is against this background that the surgery of rectal cancer will be discussed.

Choice of procedure

There are today three main categories of potentially curative surgery for rectal cancer:

1. Anterior resection with or without a colo-anal pouch: the radical removal of the involved segment of bowel with subsequent anastomosis.
2. Abdominoperineal excision: the Miles operation mentioned above.
3. Local excision: 'simple' removal via the anus of the disc of rectal wall harbouring the tumour.

The choice of operation depends to a variable degree on a series of factors, including:

• the size, site and apparent degree of advancement of the tumour;
• the patient's general condition, age and physical stature;
• the patient's and surgeon's preferences.

The choice is in some cases obvious – the high, small cancer in a fit man will usually be treated by anterior resection, while for the very low, bulky, aggressive tumour, particularly in the unfit or obese man, Miles' procedure is the obvious operation. A small proportion (around 5 per cent) of small, early tumours close to the anus may be suitable for transanal local excision (Killingback 1985, Morson 1985, Whiteway et al 1985). In many cases, however, the choice of procedure is less clear cut and much more likely to depend on the surgeon's experience and inclinations.

Description of the procedures

The two radical approaches, anterior resection and Miles' operation, are major abdominal procedures, requiring all the usual preparations and precautions. In both, a long midline incision is necessary, followed by careful abdominal assessment to check for spread to other organs.

Anterior resection

The left side of the colon is mobilized to allow its delivery into the pelvis for anastomosis to the distal bowel end after the excision of the affected segment. The rectum is then mobilized, keeping it in a clearly defined plane of dissection around it and its investing mesorectum, the fatty tissue lying mainly behind the rectum, which contains its blood supply and lymphatic drainage. Particular care has to be taken to avoid injury to the autonomic nerves lying immediately behind the upper third of the mesorectum and the sides, and in front of the lower two-thirds of the rectum; it appears, at least in terms of sexual morbidity, that men are more at risk than women in this element of the dissection.

The dissection is taken down to a level 3–5 cm below the level of tumour, at which point the rectum and mesorectum are transected. Depending on the level of the tumour and the technical difficulty of the operation, the level of the transection may lie anywhere down to the top end of the anal canal.

Having removed the involved segment and the tissues containing its lymphatic drainage, the surgeon will decide whether to make an end-to-end anastomosis or fashion a colonic pouch (see Chapter 6). The anastomosis is made either by the traditional hand-sutured technique or by using a stapling device inserted through the anus.

Depending on a series of factors, including the level of the anastomosis above the anus, the technical difficulty of the procedure and the general state of the patient, the surgeon must decide whether to finish the operation at that point or to 'defunction' the rectum, i.e. make a temporary colostomy or ileostomy upstream of the anastomosis to optimize the chance of healing and to avoid complications, particularly leakage of the anastomosis in the immediate postoperative period.

Abdominoperineal excision

This operation requires two surgical approaches: transabdominal and perineal. The operation includes the same abdominal dissection as occurs in anterior resection, extending all the way to the muscular pelvic floor. At the same time, or immediately afterwards, the surgeon makes an incision around the anus, which is extended upwards to the pelvic floor; the latter is then cut circumferentially, thus meeting up with the abdominal dissection and allowing the rectum to be removed through the perineum. The operation finishes with the formation of a colostomy in the left lower quadrant of the abdomen, after which the abdomen and perineum are closed.

Local excision

This procedure can usually be employed only if the tumour is lying within easy reach via the anus, for example within 6–7 cm of the anus. The operation is performed with the patient lying in the position that gives the surgeon the best access in that particular case, either in the lithotomy position (patients lying on their back with their legs held flexed and apart in stirrups attached to the operating table) or the prone position (on their front, with their legs apart on padded leg supports).

A self-retaining retractor is placed in the anus, and a dilute epinephrine solution is injected through the rectal wall to minimize bleeding. A disc of rectal wall is defined and excised by diathermy or scissor dissection, the defect being closed with sutures. The specimen is then examined in detail by the pathologist to check that it has been completely excised, that it has not penetrated beyond the outer surface of the muscular bowel wall and that it has a histological pattern less aggressive than 'poorly differentiated'. Should the tumour 'fail' on any of these counts, the patient should be advised that the risk of recurrence is greater than preoperatively predicted and that one of the radical operations described above is needed.

Tumours situated higher in the rectum that otherwise fulfil the criteria for possible transanal excision can be removed using a technique called transanal endoscopic microsurgery, in which a 4 cm diameter airtight operating proctoscope is inserted; through this, the tumour can be excised from the inflated rectum under binocular vision, using a series of special dissecting and suturing instruments (Buess et al 1992).

Morbidity of rectal cancer surgery

Perhaps more than in any other non-genital cancer surgery, that for rectal cancer harbours significant risks for sexual and bladder function in men (it appearing, for some reason, that women are at less risk of manifesting such morbidity). The nerve supply to the organs of sexual function and to the bladder lies in close proximity to the planes of surgical dissection; this comprises the sympathetic nerves in the hypogastric plexus and the sacral parasympathetic supply in the nervi erigentes (Scholefield & Northover 1995). Damage to the former may result in disorders of bladder emptying, while the latter are responsible for penile erection and ejaculation.

Until relatively recently, many surgeons were fatalistic about such nerve damage: rectal cancer surgery was seen as carrying an almost inevitable risk of urinary problems and impotence – in up to 50 per cent of cases in some reports. In recent times, as the anatomy of the nerves has been better understood and as the pattern of dissection and the methods of achieving it have been refined, morbidity has fallen dramatically.

Unless the nerves are actually invaded by the tumour, or the anatomy of the patient is such to make visualization very difficult, it is usually possible to avoid such complications. Damage to these nerves may be partial or complete, in terms of both the anatomy of the injury and the extent of functional deficit. If the injury does occur, it is unlikely to recover completely.

Adjuvant therapy

Overall, surgery alone is curative in around 60 per cent of those rectal cancer cases in which a radical operation is performed. Although an improvement in outcome may be made possible by an improvement in surgical technique, most efforts to increase the cure rate have been directed towards adjuvant therapy, that is the addition to surgery of radiotherapy, chemotherapy or immunotherapy (alone or in various combinations), before, during or after the operation.

There can today be no doubt that at least some forms of adjuvant therapy can improve the outlook in this disease, although which patients are most likely to benefit, and which modes or regimens of treatment – and in which combinations – are best, remain matters of hot debate and widespread clinical research. Radiotherapy is essentially a locoregional modality, aimed mainly at reducing the risk of local cancer recurrence in rectal cancer cases, whilst chemotherapy, albeit probably adding to the local efficacy of radiotherapy, is seen mainly as a means of improving the chance of survival through its systemic effect.

Treatment modalities

Radiotherapy

This may be delivered pre- or postoperatively, whilst in a few centres it can be delivered to the precise site at risk of recurrence with the abdomen open at operation. Given preoperatively, it can be seen in randomized trials to 'downstage' the tumour (i.e. to cause the tumour to revert to an apparently more favourable pathological stage) (Medical Research Council Rectal Cancer Working Party 1996, Graf et al 1997). Regimens range from high-dose therapy (in the region of a total dose of 4,000–5,000 cGy, delivered over a 4–5 week period, followed by a 6 week rest prior to surgery) to lower-dose, rapid courses (1,000–2,500 cGy in the week immediately prior to surgery) (Swedish Rectal Cancer Group 1997).

The major disadvantages of preoperative therapy include the delay in operating if radical radiotherapy is used and the blanket delivery of therapy to all cases in the absence of pathological staging information, which might allow its more selective use. Its advantages include a lesser likelihood of radiation morbidity, particularly damage to the small intestine.

Postoperative radiotherapy does not delay operation and can be withheld from those patients who, on pathological examination of their operative specimens, can be predicted to be highly likely to have been cured by surgery alone (Medical Research Council Rectal Cancer Working Party 1996). The most important disadvantage of postoperative therapy is small bowel radiation damage, made more probable by operation-induced adhesions, which cause the small bowel inevitably to be held in the field of treatment. This leads to significant morbidity and, in around 5 per cent of cases, occasional mortality.

There are no widely accepted guidelines for adjuvant therapy in rectal cancer, so practice differs widely. Most surgeons would accept that, in cases of locally advanced rectal cancer, in which the feasibility of surgical clearance appears to be marginal, preoperative radiotherapy is advisable. Recent trials have amplified this contention. Many surgeons, particularly those whose local recurrence rate is favourably low, prefer to reserve adjuvant radiotherapy for those patients in whom the pathological examination of the surgical specimen suggests a particular risk of recurrence; this group therefore favours a selective policy of postoperative therapy.

Recent trials in Sweden have yielded persuasive evidence for the uniform use of short-course preoperative therapy, having demonstrated a decrease in local recurrence at all pathological stages, even the earliest (Swedish Rectal Cancer Group 1997). This debate will undoubtedly continue.

Chemotherapy

Adjuvant chemotherapy for rectal cancer has been investigated for more than 40 years and has mainly involved the use of 5-fluorouracil, either alone or in combination with other drugs. Until 10 years ago, the results were uniformly quite disappointing, but since the late 1980s, trials have shown promise, leading to a much wider use of adjuvant chemotherapy. Opinions differ on its role in various clinical situations, but the evidence for its efficacy is sufficient for it to be seen, particularly by American oncologists, as uniformly relevant therapy in the majority of cases.

In rectal cancer, chemotherapy may be used alone or in combination with radiotherapy. Again, trials in the early 1990s led to advice in the USA for the uniform use of combination therapy (radiotherapy and chemotherapy together), at least in stage C tumours (Krook et al 1991), although many European commentators have again not found the evidence sufficiently persuasive. Evidence from the Mayo Clinic indicates strongly that more patients are likely to suffer significant side-effects of adjuvant therapy than will benefit.

Postoperative follow-up

It has become a convention that colorectal cancer patients are 'followed up' for 5 years after surgery. A majority of surgeons aim to see their patients 3 monthly for the first 2 years and 6 monthly thereafter until 5 years postsurgery, then discharging the patient from further surveillance. This is based on two tenets: that the majority of the risk of recurrence has dissipated by the end of 2 years and that survival becomes parallel to that of the general population (the risk of recurrence having disappeared) at 5 years.

The process of follow-up after cancer surgery has several aims (Cochrane et al 1980):

- to identify postoperative complications;
- to reassure the patient;
- to allow an audit of the surgeon's performance;
- to detect metachronous tumours;
- to detect recurrent cancer.

Most postoperative complications, except perhaps incisional hernia, manifest themselves within the first year. Many patients are alarmed rather than reassured by an impending outpatient follow-up visit, and few surgeons make proper use of follow-up data to review, criticize and alter their cancer management strategies. In addition, only around 5 per cent of bowel cancer patients develop metachronous cancer. Thus, on the face of it, the detection of recurrent cancer should carry some promise, at least for some patients, that early diagnosis will lead to an improved prospect of cure of recurrence. In other words, to quote Moertel et al (1978), 'the only outcome for most patients would seem to be the needless anxiety produced by premature knowledge of the presence of a fatal disease'.

There is currently no evidence that any particular pattern of follow-up surveillance, from the most frequent, invasive and expensive to the least so – merely telling patients about the symptoms of recurrence after recovery from surgery and asking them to make contact if such symptoms occur – has any advantage in terms of survivability of recurrent colorectal cancer (Virgo et al 1995).

Reflecting the high cost and low evidence of the effectiveness of bowel cancer follow-up, the UK government's National Health Service Executive recently published recommendations that appropriately reflect the difficult and evolving balance between the advantages of postoperative vigilance and the costs – financial, emotional and physical – of surveillance and consequent interventions (Haward 1997).

Follow-up procedures

Despite the foregoing critique of the follow-up process, most patients can expect some or all of the following procedures during the years following their treatment:

- *Clinical assessment.* This is likely to be offered following the timetable mentioned above. It will include questioning with regard to symptoms, general physical examination and, particularly after rectal cancer surgery, rigid sigmoidoscopic examination.
- *Colonoscopy.* This should have been performed perioperatively to exclude a synchronous second primary cancer and/or associated adenomata. Depending on the presence of association neoplasia, the age of the patient and the enthusiasm of the clinician, repeated colonoscopy may be offered every 0–5 years in perpetuity after primary treatment.
- *Scanning procedures.* As the liver is the most frequently affected distant site of metastasis, examination may be performed using US, CT or MR scanning, particularly in the first 2 or 3 years after surgery. The possibility of cure by the resection of localized liver recurrence is quite high – in the region of 30 per cent (Hughes et

al 1988) – but whether presymptomatic diagnosis by regular scanning increases the proportion thus cured remains another area of
debate in the controversy surrounding follow-up practice.

*   *Serum marker assay.* Although frequent blood sampling for carci-
    noembryoninc antigen is widely practised, particularly in the
    USA, there is yet again no evidence of efficacy in this field;
    indeed, preliminary data from the only randomized trial in this
    area strongly indicate no survival benefit (Northover 1995).

It may well be that, in resource-conscious health-care
programmes such as the that of UK National Health Service, rigid
follow-up regimens that consume precious funds without evidence of
benefit will be further discouraged in the immediate future (Haward
1997).

Prognosis

Although the surgeon is often able to identify incurable distant or
local spread at the time of presentation, the pathologist is, in cases in
which a surgical attempt at cure has been made, the person able to
give the most important information on prognosis (Quirke et al
1986, Jass et al 1987). Although there is much information to be
gained from careful pathological examination, many pathologists
still fail to make an adequate assessment. For this to be achieved, at
least the following must be examined:

*   *Depth of invasion by the primary tumour.* Has it spread through the full
    thickness of the muscle wall of the bowel? If it has, does it reach to
    the radical resection margin (implying that some of the tumour
    may have been left behind)?
*   *Lymph node involvement.* The nodes draining the tumour must be
    dissected out individually, counted and examined for the pres-
    ence of tumour.
*   *Differentiation of the tumour.* This may vary between different parts of
    the primary tumour and in any involved nodes; the area of worst
    differentiation should be used to provide prognostic information.

On the basis of this information, the pathologist is able to stage the
tumour, using the Dukes staging system or a variation of it.

The classical Dukes staging system (Figure 3.2) and its various modifications spawned over the decades since it was first described leave much to be desired. The breadwinner, for example, needing to plan for the future who is told that his tumour is at Dukes stage B could almost as usefully have a coin tossed on his behalf when trying to divine his chance of survival.

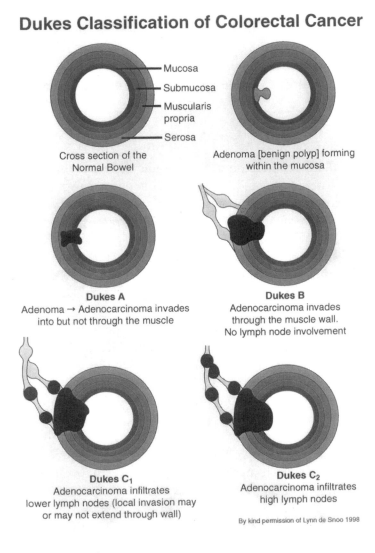

Figure 3.2 Dukes staging.

Prevention

As such a large proportion of bowel cancer risk appears to be associated with dietary and other environmental/lifestyle factors, a corresponding proportion of cases ought to be preventable by suitable alterations in diet and lifestyle. In order to provide evidence upon which to base dietary advice, various randomized controlled trials (RCTs) have been or are being performed. Because of the relative rarity of bowel cancer in the general population (its prevalence being approximately 1 in 500 at any one time), and despite its prominence in the league table of killing cancers, RCTs using cancer incidence or mortality as the end-point are, in practical terms, very difficult to design or perform; instead adenoma incidence or recurrence has generally been used as a measure of effect.

The Women's Health Initiative in the USA, involving 63,000 randomized subjects, is the biggest study using cancer itself as the measured end-point (Roussoux et al 1995); evidence should become available within the next decade upon which to develop dietary preventative advice – applicable to men as well as women!

Screening

Screening is the process by which asymptomatic individuals are offered an intervention, which may indicate that they are at increased risk of the target disease and hence need more invasive investigation to exclude or confirm this. For screening to be considered worthwhile as a public health measure used as part of the overall strategy for coping with a particular condition, several criteria must be met:

- The condition must be sufficiently common, with the potential for intervention earlier in its natural history to alter the outcome favourably.
- The test must be safe, cheap and acceptable to the target population, easy to apply and sufficiently sensitive and specific.
- There must be an infrastructure capable of coping with the management of all those found to have positive screening test results.

The first two of these criteria has been broadly seen to be fulfilled in colorectal cancer, although a clear view of the effect on the incidence and mortality effect required the performance of large RCTs. In the UK and in many other countries, the endoscopy and radiological services currently available would not cope with the load generated by nationwide screening. Only in Germany has there been a national policy of bowel cancer screening (despite a deficient evidence base, and generating poor population compliance, particularly amongst men); as data from RCTs have become available in the past few years, other countries, including the UK, are seriously contemplating the issue.

Screening methods

Two main approaches have been investigated:

- tests looking for tumour products in the stool, principally occult blood (Greegor 1971) and more recently mutated genes in shed cancer cells (Sidransky et al 1992);
- direct examination of the bowel mucosa using endoscopes, particularly the flexible sigmoidoscope (Atkin et al 1993, Selby et al 1992, Verne et al 1996) but also the colonoscope (Lieberman & Smith 1991).

Stool tests

Faecal occult blood tests (FOBTs) have been the subject of intensive investigation for more than two decades. They work on the principle that colorectal tumours, cancers more than adenomas, bleed intermittently, often without the blood being sufficient to be visible.

The most widely investigated FOBT, Haemoccult®, relies on the presence in the stool of haematin, which, on reaction with hydrogen peroxide, turns the indicator substance, guaiac, blue (Greegor 1971). The person being screened provides a faecal sample on a commercially produced card infiltrated with guaiac, the card being sent to a laboratory, where hydrogen peroxide is applied. Two samples from each of three stools are tested. If the test is positive, there is an approximately 10 per cent chance that the person is suffering from bowel cancer; a colonoscopy or barium enema examination is then required to exclude a tumour.

False-positive results can occur from the presence of an alternative bleeding lesion (such as piles, diverticular disease or an upper gastrointestinal bleeding lesion, or arising from medication such as aspirin) or the ingestion of animal blood in food or certain foodstuffs, which can trigger a peroxidase reaction. Conversely, rectal cancers are more likely than colonic cancers to be falsely negative, as the disruption of the red cells, leading to the release of haemoglobin, is necessary to produce a positive result; in rectal cancer cases, the bleeding is often fresh, and hence the red cells more uniformly intact, thus triggering a positive FOBT.

If investigation resulting from a positive FOBT, either a colonoscopy or a double-contrast barium enema, shows a cancer to be present, there is a high probability that it will be at a pathologically early stage and hence amenable to curative treatment.

Results from RCTs performed in Minnesota, Denmark and the UK have been published in the past few years; they indicate that a decrease in mortality of 15–30 per cent might be achieved through the introduction of national FOBT screening (Hardcastle et al 1996). In the UK, pilot centres to test the wider implementation of such a programme have been chosen and will soon begin screening.

Endoscopic screening

Two tests have been investigated: flexible sigmoidoscopy, which can examine only the left colon and rectum, and colonoscopy, with the capacity to reach the whole large bowel. The obvious advantages of endoscopic screening are the ability to examine the bowel mucosa directly and to be able to remove adenomas or polypoid malignancies at the time of the screening examination (Lieberman & Smith 1991); on the other hand, the screening intervention is more complex and potentially injurious, thereby being perhaps less likely to encourage compliance from the target population. Studies have nevertheless shown the use of flexible sigmoidoscopy to be acceptable, safe and effective in detection (Verne et al 1996).

Although it is a less extensive procedure, flexible sigmoidoscopy can reach the segment most at risk of the development of neoplasia, being quicker, safer and less expensive. Those found to have 'high-risk' (large, villous or multiple) adenomas at flexible sigmoidoscopy can be referred for colonoscopy (Atkin et al 1993). A large RCT in the UK is currently examining the efficacy of flexible sigmoidoscopy, and a similar investigation of colonoscopy is underway in the USA.

High-risk groups

Although bowel cancer is a common condition, there are some who are at even higher risk of this disease, primarily those with an inheritable predisposition and those with long-standing extensive ulcerative colitis.

Inherited predisposition

There are two principal dominantly inheritable conditions, familial adenomatous polyposis (FAP) and hereditary non-polyposis colorectal cancer syndrome (HNPCC). Both are rare, accounting for no more than 5 per cent of all bowel cancers between them. Neither condition is gender linked, nor is there any evidence of significant geographical variation.

Familial adenomatous polyposis

This condition is characterized by the development in the teenage years of hundreds or thousands of adenomas on the colorectal mucosa, some of which progress to malignancy by the age of 40 years if they are left untreated (Bussey 1975). Associated lesions in affected individuals include duodenal adenomas, desmoid tumours, mainly affecting the abdomen, and various incidental abnormalities such as benign osteomas, skin cysts and retinal pigmentation. The condition is caused by mutations in a gene on the long arm (5q) of chromosome 5 (Bodmer et al 1987, Leppert et al 1987). Cancer-preventative, prophylactic, sphincter-preserving surgery, removing the bulk of the large intestine, is carried out in the mid to late teens for affected individuals (Bussey 1975).

Hereditary non-polyposis colorectal cancer syndrome

This condition produces a less obvious clinical picture in affected individuals: there is no carpet of adenomas to betray the diagnosis. There is a predilection for right-sided tumours, occurring at a younger average age, and more frequently with multiple primary tumours in affected families (Lynch et al 1985).

The condition is caused by mutations in the mismatch repair genes that 'police' the process of cell division, usually identifying and rectifying chance mutations in the genome (Bronner et al

1994, Parsons et al 1993). The resulting inefficiency in the process leads to the accumulation of the somatic mutations that underlie the ACS. The identification of families harbouring this condition allows them to be offered regular colonoscopic surveillance so that adenomas can be removed, preventing their progression to frank malignancy.

Non-FAP, non-HNPCC familial cancer

There are some families who appear to harbour an inheritable risk who do not appear to have the currently understood predisposing mutations. If a family pedigree gives rise to sufficient suspicion of a predisposition, even in the absence of an identified genetic explanation, colonoscopic surveillance should be offered (Hodgson et al 1995).

Inflammatory bowel disease

Colorectal cancer occurs more frequently in patients with ulcerative colitis or Crohn's disease than amongst the general population. The cancer risk is small in Crohn's patients and in those with anatomically limited or recent-onset ulcerative colitis. In those who have had ulcerative colitis for 10 years or more, and in whom the disease affects the majority of the large bowel, the risk of cancer rises sharply. In those with extensive colitis lsting for over 20 years, the cancer risk exceeds 20 per cent.

Cancer is usually preceded by the development of dysplastic mucosal lesions; regular (1–2 yearly) colonoscopy to try to identify these premalignant lesions may lead to effective preventative surgical treatment, but the debate over the efficacy of such surveillance programmes continues (Gage 1986, Rutegard et al 1988).

The future

Rectal cancer often poses enormous difficulties in management; although great strides have been made in minimizing surgical mutilation, the death rate for the disease has hardly changed in decades. In the immediate future, we must look to screening to direct treatment to the early stages of the disease, when surgery is at its most effective.

Improved adjuvant therapy – making use of our growing understanding of the molecular biology of the disease – shows signs of
imminent influence, but the real challenge is the development of a
sufficient understanding of the mechanisms of inception and
progression of this tumour. When this has reached a stage at which
risk factors and aetiological pathways can be altered, we will begin to
see rectal cancer losing its major role as a cause of death and debility
in our society.

Patient/family support network

Family and friends provide vital support for a person with cancer:
social support is critical for individuals coping with any major life
event such as the diagnosis of cancer (Lackner et al 1994, Ell et al
1989).

Cancer is never experienced in isolation. The impact of the
patients' disease and treatment is also felt by the people who make
up their support system, who are expected to offer support and
respond positively. Caring for people with cancer is stressful (Dunkel-
Schetter 1984); key carers will feel more able to provide help and
support to the patient if they themselves feel involved, informed and
supported.

Outside the family and friends network, support is available from
a range of professionals. Macmillan nurses specialize in cancer care,
working either in the hospital or in the home. Their support is aimed
at facilitating the adjustment of the individual and his family to the
cancer diagnosis and its effects. Macmillan nurses are often involved
from time of diagnosis and will take referrals from patients and/or
relatives.

Working alongside health-care professionals, many voluntary organizations exist to help people with cancer. They generally also offer
emotional support and practical help to carers. One example is
CancerBACUP (see Useful Addresses), which has a cancer information service, a free counselling service and a series of patient booklets.
Their booklet *Understanding cancer of the colon and rectum* offers useful
supplementary written information to patients diagnosed with colorectal cancer. There are currently two national charities concerned solely
with colorectal cancer – Colon Cancer Concern and the Crocus Trust
– both providing written information and telephone access.

Local branches of national organizations often exist, aimed at providing the ongoing personalized support that may provide patients with the confidence and direction they need to address the problems that this disease can bring (Evans 1995). Cancerlink has over 600 cancer support and self-help groups nationwide and offers a helpline in many different languages. For those patients with or anticipating a stoma, the British Colostomy Association and the Ileostomy and Internal Pouch Support Group offer local contacts.

CHAPTER 4

The ileo-anal pouch

R.J. NICHOLLS AND JULIA WILLIAMS

Historical development of surgery

Ulcerative colitis was first defined as a clinico-pathological entity in the late nineteenth century. In the past 100 years, medical and surgical treatment have considerably advanced. The first operation to be used was appendicostomy, in which the appendix was brought out onto the anterior abdominal wall as a small stoma, which was then used to introduce therapeutic solutions as a topical treatment to the inflamed large bowel. The mortality with this procedure was, however, over 50 per cent, and its effectiveness was doubtful.

In 1913, Brown first used a loop ileostomy to defunction the large bowel, and although the mortality was again very high, discernible clinical improvement, sometimes dramatic, was observed in a number of cases. By the 1920s, ileorectal bypass procedures were being introduced, but surgeons were still so fearful of a high mortality that resection of the inflamed large bowel was considered to be too dangerous. In the 1940s, Miller and colleagues in Canada described a series of patients with ulcerative colitis who were treated by resection of the colon with ileostomy. There was no mortality in the 24 patients reported.

The appreciation that surgery is effective when the disease is removed may seem simple to us now, but it took many decades to be realised. This advance marks the modern era of surgery for ulcerative colitis. Colectomy was followed by conventional proctocolectomy, which became the standard operation after Brooke (1952) had developed the everted spout ileostomy, making life so much easier for the ostomist.

A permanent ileostomy was, however, perceived by some surgeons and many patients to be a disadvantage, and the subsequent story of how surgery for ulcerative colitis evolved was directed towards stoma avoidance. Thus, colectomy with ileorectal anastomosis had enthusiastic advocates in the 1950s (Aylett 1953), although others felt strongly that this operation should not be undertaken since the patient was left with a rectum constantly at risk of the development of cancer.

Whereas many patients had a satisfactory outcome after colectomy with ileorectal anastomosis, others did not, chiefly owing to persisting inflammation within the rectum. Reports in the literature have shown a highly variable outcome after this operation. Failure, defined as the need for proctectomy with permanent ileostomy, ranges from 10 per cent to over 40 per cent in patients followed for 5 years or more (Aylett 1966, Hawley 1988).

Colectomy with ileorectal anastomosis is a compromise procedure since it leaves part of the diseased rectum, its only justification being the avoidance of a permanent ileostomy. Failure largely arises from the persisting disease, either because its inflammatory manifestations compromise function or because of malignant transformation. In Aylett's large series of patients, a subsequent occurrence of carcinoma in the rectum occurred in about 5 per cent (Baker et al 1978), the tumours often being advanced.

Restorative proctocolectomy

If conventional proctocolectomy removes all the inflamed tissue at the price of a permanent ileostomy, and colectomy with ileorectal anastomosis avoids an ileostomy but renders the patient still susceptible to the disease, then restorative proctocolectomy has the merit of avoiding each disadvantage by a total removal of the disease with sphincter preservation.

The first proctocolectomy with ileo-anal anastomosis was carried out by Ravitch & Sabiston (1947). They used it for familial adenomatous polyposis (FAP), but, shortly afterwards, the operation was also employed for ulcerative colitis. Valiente & Bacon (1955) reviewed the literature of reports of the so-called 'straight ileo-anal anastomosis' and concluded that the functional result was poor. This was mainly due to the frequency, and particularly urgency, of defaecation. These authors were the first to suggest that the inclusion of a reservoir into the ileo-anal reconstruction might improve function. Such procedures were performed on dogs, but their high mortality prevented the application to humans at that time.

In the 1960s, Kock (1969) reported the use of an ileal reservoir designed to employ an internal valve as a means of creating a continent ileostomy. Although this was still an abdominal stoma, the technique demonstrated that a small bowel reservoir could be readily tolerated by the patient and also that quality of life was greatly improved in those patients who had a successful outcome. This operation is now performed much less often owing to the introduction of restorative proctocolectomy. There are, however, many reports in the literature of the Kock operation (Hulten et al 1988), all of which show a significant incidence of valve failure, ranging from 10 per cent to over 40 per cent. This complication requires revision at a subsequent operation (see Chapter 5).

In the early 1970s, Sir Alan Parks combined many of the advantages of these previous surgical developments to create the modern restorative proctocolectomy. By the surgical removal of the colon, the rectum and the mucosa of the upper anal canal, the diseased tissue was removed. By preserving the anal sphincter, continent anal function was possible. Adding a small bowel reservoir and bringing this to the anus improved function compared with a 'straight' ileo-anal anastomosis. These goals have to a large extent been fulfilled in the majority of patients undergoing this operation.

Restorative proctocolectomy has gone through several modifications since it was first described in 1978 (Parks & Nicholls 1978), but the basic principles have remained the same. There have, however, been changes, including alterations in the method of rectal dissection, the type of reservoir, the technique of ileo-anal anastomosis and whether a mucosectomy should or should not be carried out. The need for a defunctioning temporary stoma has also been questioned. Along with this natural evolution, the results of the procedure in terms of failure, complications, function and long-term consequences have now been well defined.

General indications for surgery in ulcerative colitis

The indications for surgery in ulcerative colitis are threefold: a failure of medical treatment, a failure of growth in a child and neoplastic transformation. This last indication occurs at a cumulative rate of about 1 per cent per year, starting around 10 years after the onset of the disease. Thus, by 20 years, 10 per cent of a colitic population will have developed a carcinoma. There is some evidence that this rate increases beyond 30 years from diagnosis, which is relevant since colitis is a disease of young people.

The failure of medical treatment is manifest is several ways, including chronic unremitting disease, recurrent acute exacerbations, poor function (particularly frequency and urgency), extra-alimentary manifestations and steroid dependence. A decision to recommend surgery requires experience on the part of the physician or surgeon and must involve the patient fully in the discussion.

Acutely ill patients and those who have toxic dilatation or colonic perforation should, however, have a colectomy with ileostomy and preservation of the rectal stump. This procedure may also be the most suitable option for those on a high dose of steroids and those in whom the diagnosis of ulcerative colitis is uncertain (Parker & Nicholls 1992). Patients undergoing this operation can then have a restorative proctectomy as a second stage provided that they fulfil the criteria listed below.

General indications for surgery in FAP

Owing to the nature of the disease, a very high average number of adenomas is present in the large bowel of a person with FAP, and, because every adenoma has malignant potential, major prophylactic surgery is justified. Surgeons still, however, debate which surgical option – ileorectal anastomosis or restorative proctocolectomy – is more appropriate for the patient. A restorative proctocolectomy is normally recommended for patients with a higher risk of developing rectal cancer or those who present with malignancy high in the rectum.

The functional results of restorative proctocolectomy are similar to those of ileorectal anastomosis, but the morbidity rate is higher in restorative proctocolectomy. In addition, lifelong follow-up is recommended. This is because of the risk of other cancers and also because it provides an opportunity to ensure contact with the rest of the family. In doing so, the next generation will be more likely to be screened at puberty and hence avoid colorectal cancer.

Choice of elective procedure

Having decided on surgery, there are three elective options available to the patient:

- Conventional proctocolectomy with permanent ileostomy (Figure 4.1).
- Colectomy with ileorectal anastomosis (Figure 4.2).
- Restorative proctocolectomy (Figure 4.3).

The final choice will depend on a combination of medical factors and patient preference. Conventional proctocolectomy may well be preferred by some patients on being fully informed of the potential disadvantages of restorative procedures. They may prefer a simple, one-stage operation with a low prospect of complications and a short

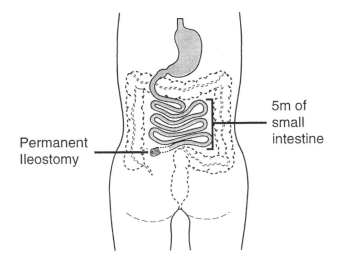

Figure 4.1 Conventional proctocolectomy with permanent ileostomy.

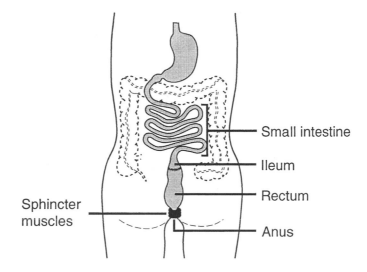

Small intestine

Ileum

Rectum

Sphincter
muscles

Anus

Figure 4.2 Ileorectal anastomosis.

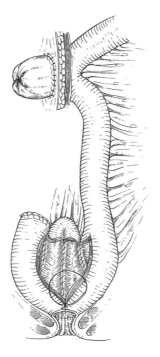

Figure 4.3 Restorative proctocolectomy, illustrating a 'W' pouch.

timescale of recovery as being the acceptable price of a permanent ileostomy. Others, however, will strongly resist an ileostomy, and this is the only reason for considering the other two options.

Colectomy with ileorectal anastomosis possesses the disadvantages outlined above. In current practice, this operation is suitable only when the rectum is relatively non-inflamed and expansible with no evidence of neoplastic transformation (dysplasia), and provided that the anal sphincter is competent (Baker et al 1978). Twenty years ago, when restorative proctocolectomy was first introduced, about 20–30 per cent of patients in most specialist units underwent colectomy with ileorectal anastomosis. Today, the proportion has fallen dramatically to below 10 per cent because of the greater use of restorative proctocolectomy in patients who would previously have had an ileorectal anastomosis.

The choice of surgical procedure has in many ways changed over the past 20 years, as seen in Figure 4.4; this is mainly because of improved surgical techniques, a different outlook on the long-term outcome of surgery and an increased appreciation of improving quality of life.

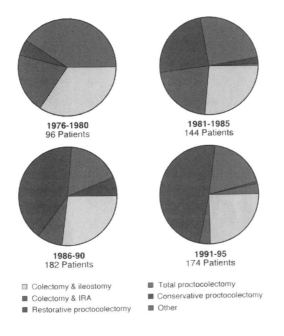

Figure 4.4 Elective operations: surgery for ulcerative colitis, 1976–1995.

Indications for restorative proctocolectomy

Crohn's disease

Restorative proctocolectomy is contraindicated in the following circumstances. Although it has been suggested that patients with Crohn's disease can be treated successfully by this operation, with a low failure rate (Panis et al 1996), the experience of almost all other units has been that Crohn's disease results in failure in a high proportion of patients. Thus, a failure rate of 40 per cent or more over a few years' follow-up has been reported. It is highly likely that this proportion will increase as the length of follow-up extends.

Most of the experience of restorative proctocolectomy from Crohn's disease has derived from the use of the operation in a patient erroneously believed to have had ulcerative colitis. Panis et al (1996) were careful to define the type of Crohn's disease they felt to be suitable. These were patients with inflammation of the colon and rectum with anal sparing. This combination is not common in clinical practice, since 70 per cent or more of patients with Crohn's proctitis have an anal lesion. Most surgeons feel that restorative proctocolectomy is contraindicated in Crohn's disease.

Indeterminate colitis

There is a group of patients with inflammatory bowel disease in whom the histopathologists cannot distinguish between ulcerative colitis and Crohn's disease. This situation is referred to as indeterminate colitis. Indeterminate colitis is not a disease; it is simply a convenient label for the 10 per cent or so of patients with inflammatory bowel disease who cannot readily be diagnosed as having ulcerative colitis on the one hand or Crohn's disease on the other (Nicholls & Wells 1992). It most often arises on pathological examination of the colon after emergency removal in the severely ill patient. Here the severity of inflammation may destroy some of the characteristic features that allow the pathologist to distinguish between the two.

Given a pathological report of 'indeterminate colitis', the clinician should take more biopsies (the rectum usually still being present), examine the small intestine using contrast radiology and examine the anus carefully for lesions that will increase the likelihood that the patient is in fact suffering from Crohn's disease.

Further investigation is likely to reduce the number of patients in this category, but there will still be a residuum in whom it is truly impossible to distinguish.

In these, restorative proctocolectomy would appear to offer almost as good a result as is seen patients with unequivocal ulcerative colitis (Nicholls 1984), although there is some evidence that the failure rate may be higher in indeterminate colitis (Hyman et al 1991). It is evident that the histopathologist has a vital role in accurate diagnosis. Expertise is variable, but in most units, the occurrence of a false-positive diagnosis of ulcerative colitis is well below 5 per cent of cases.

Other considerations

Restorative proctocolectomy should not be undertaken in patients with an incompetent anal sphincter. This must be assessed preoperatively, and, where available, tests of anorectal physiology should be carried out. Clinical examination and manometry will reveal an incompetent anal sphincter.

Patients who are severely ill as described above should have an initial colectomy with ileostomy before a restorative proctocolectomy. It is wise to allow an interval of at least 4 months between these two procedures.

Occasionally, a patient with ulcerative colitis or FAP will present with an already established carcinoma. Provided that there is no dissemination, and provided also that surgical clearance will be adequate accordingly to current concepts of cancer surgery, it is reasonable to advise a restorative proctocolectomy. Patients with a carcinoma in the low rectum should, however, have a conventional proctocolectomy.

The incidence of pouchitis in patients with sclerosing cholangitis is much higher than in those without, a rate of over 50 per cent having been reported (Pincowsky & Ekbom 1995). It is unwise therefore to consider a restorative proctocolectomy in the patient with sclerosing cholangitis.

Patient choice

The second component to deciding on the choice of operation is the patient's own particular desire. Many patients are extremely well informed, but those who are not should be given a full account of the advantages and disadvantages of each option, along with the probable incidence of complications and failure, the functional outcome and the long-term prospects. This information should be supported with appropriate written health education material.

Patients should also be given the opportunity to meet others who have already had such surgery and be put in touch with patient support groups. It is important to note that each individual who has undergone a restorative procedure has been exposed to a unique set of circumstances, so, in order to provide a balance when making the choice of surgical procedure, potential pouch owners should meet with others who have had both good and bad experiences.

Many patients express difficulty in choosing a surgical option, and it is therefore extremely important for the nurse specialist to assist in this decision-making process. It is the patients who must ultimately make the decision of which surgical option they will take, but emphasis must be given to the strengths and coping mechanisms of individuals in order for them to make a rational decision.

Surgical technique

A full bowel preparation is not felt to be necessary, but the patient should take clear liquids for 24–48 hours preoperatively. It is important to check the haemoglobin level and to have blood cross-matched for transfusion. Anti-embolism therapy is likely to be commenced in the immediate postoperative period.

Patients undergoing the first stage of the restorative procedure will require the siting of the stoma. Even though the stoma is deemed temporary, it is important that it is sited appropriately (Table 4.1). For patients who have experienced an ileostomy before, it is probable that the original site will be used. A new site is necessary only at the patient's request or as a consequence of the surgery, for example the inability to mobilize enough small bowel so that the stoma is not created under tension.

The operation

The patient is fully anaesthetized and placed in the Lloyd-Davis position, the hips and knees each being flexed to about 120°. This (Figure 6.3, p. 123) allows simultaneous access to the abdomen and

Table 4.1 Key points when siting a stoma

- The potential site must be visible to the patient
- Avoid skin creases
- Avoid surgical scars from previous surgery and drain sites
- Avoid bony prominences
- Avoid the waist- or belt line
- Consider employment factors, for example the need to wear a seat beat for someone whose occupation is driving
- Position within the abdominal rectus sheath

---

the perineum. The bladder is catheterized and the skin prepared with an antiseptic solution. The perineal area and vagina are also cleaned. In males, the scrotum is taped to one side.

Colectomy

The abdomen is opened through a midline incision and the intra-abdominal organs carefully examined; this includes the liver, stomach, spleen and small bowel as well as the large bowel. The terminal ileum may be mildly inflamed (backwash ileitis), but evident small bowel disease should raise the possibility of Crohn's disease. Even if the right colon looks normal on the outside, as it often does, it is obligatory to perform a total colectomy.

Mobilization of the colon is begun on the right side, with early division of the bowel at the ileocaecal junction. The colon is mobilized further round the hepatic flexure along the transverse colon to the splenic flexure. There are no data available on whether the omentum should be removed or preserved. It is the author's practice to remove it as the dissection along the transverse colon proceeds. The splenic flexure is often easier to mobilize in the colitic patient since the effect of the disease, causing contraction and shortening of the colon, may bring it down within the abdomen. On mobilizing the left colon, the vessels are divided, completing the colectomy part of the procedure.

The rectal dissection

The dissection is then continued to the rectum. The sigmoid colon is mobilized to the right, and the gonadal vessels and ureter are identified and safeguarded. Dissecting more medially, the presacral nerves are identified. It is very important in patients with benign disease to preserve the pelvic autonomic nerves. Injury may lead to urinary complications as well as, more frequently, sexual dysfunction. In the male, damage to the presacral nerves results in a failure of ejaculation, and damage to the autonomic nerve plexus in the lower part of the pelvis on the lateral wall causes failure of an erection (impotence).

The use of a close rectal dissection in patients without dysplasia, and therefore without the risk of harbouring an undiagnosed cancer, avoids any chance of nerve damage. In this technique, the blood vessels entering the rectum are divided just as they do so, resulting in the removal of the rectal tube itself without any surrounding mesorectum, which remains in the patient. This is time-consuming, and many surgeons regard it as being difficult. It is nevertheless a sure way of avoiding pelvic nerve damage.

The alternative employed by most surgeons is to dissect the rectum, with its mesorectum, entering the anatomical presacral space as for a cancer dissection but identifying the presacral nerves in the upper part and staying close to the rectal wall in the lower part. In patients with dysplasia, a close rectal dissection should not be carried out since subclinical invasion (cancer) may have already developed.

The rectum is dissected downwards to the level of the pelvic floor. This will require identification of the rectovaginal and rectoprostatic septum and division of the fascia of Denonvilliers, allowing the dissection to proceed behind it. This is particularly important in the male since it avoids damage to the nerve plexuses on the back of the prostate. As the pelvic floor is approached, it is vital to avoid damage to the levator ani and puborectalis muscles.

The bowel is then divided at the level of the anorectal junction. The method of division will depend upon whether a manual or a stapled ileo-anal anastomosis is contemplated. In the former case, the bowel is simply divided at about 2 cm above the dentate line, as indicated by a perineal operator carrying out a simultaneous proctoscopy. For the latter, a transverse stapled line is placed across the rectum at the anorectal junction. It is vital that this be done at the correct level. This may be difficult to achieve in a muscular male with a narrow pelvis, but the price paid by the patient if any rectum is left behind is likely to be high.

Mobilization of the small intestine

The small intestine is then fully mobilized. The free edge of the mesentery is traced up to the duodenum, and the ileocolic artery is divided. Any intrinsic adhesions within the mesentery are also divided. Adequate mobility is essential and can easily be determined by means of a trial descent. The most mobile point on the terminal ileum is marked as the site for the future ileo-anal anastomosis.

Where the rectum has been divided, as for a manual anastomosis, a stay suture is placed on the ileum at the point selected. This is then drawn down through the anal canal by a perineal operator to deliver the small bowel through the anorectal stump. If it reaches the dentate line, it will do so after the pouch has been made. If it does not, further attempts at mobilizing the mesentery can be made until mobility is satisfactory.

Where the anal stump has been closed by a staple line, it is not possible to bring the small bowel through the anal canal, but at least a reasonable idea of mobility can be obtained by taking the point on the terminal ileum for anastomosis, a Babcocks forceps bringing that down through the pelvis to the pelvic floor.

There is much discussion on the relative merits of a manual versus a stapled anastomosis, and these will be considered in a later chapter. From a technical point of view, it is advisable to use a stapled anastomosis where the mobility of the small bowel is likely to be restricted, for example in a large male with a narrow pelvis. In other circumstances, a hand-sutured anastomosis has much to offer because it allows the surgeon to create the anastomosis at a controlled level, thus avoiding the undesirable ileal pouch–rectal anastomosis that will occur using the stapled technique if the transverse stapled line lies above the anorectal junction.

The ileal reservoir

The pouch is now constructed (Figure 4.5). Several designs have been described. The 'S' loop had the merit of adequate capacity, but the distal ileal segment between it and the ileo-anal anastomosis was responsible for a failure of spontaneous evacuation in 10–50 per cent of cases (Nicholls 1984, Rothenberger et al 1985), and the technique is therefore no longer advocated.

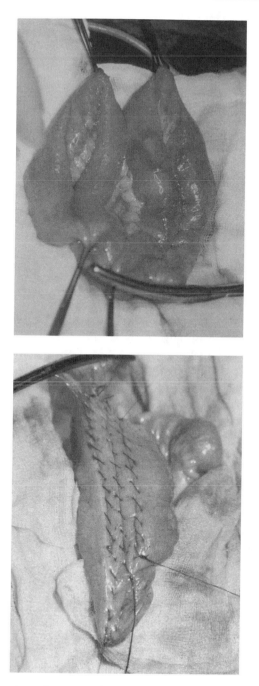

(a)

(b)

Figure 4.5 Ileo-anal pouch construction (see Plate 6 a and b).

The 'J' loop (Utsunomiya et al 1980) is simple to construct and does not have the distal ileal segment. It can be made using a stapling instrument, but its limbs should approach 20 cm in length. The 'K' pouch is based on the principle of the Kock pouch, so whereas the J pouch will be anastomosed from side to side, the K pouch will be formed from bottom to top.

The four-loop ('W') reservoir (Nicholls & Lubowski 1987) was developed in the light of the observation that the frequency of defaecation and the capacitance of the reservoir are inversely related (Pezim & Nicholls 1985a). Thus, within reason, the larger the reservoir, the lower the frequency, an observation that had also been made for the straight ileo-anal reconstruction (Heppell 1982).

The ileo-anal anastomosis

Stapled

Having completed the reservoir, the head of the circular stapler is inserted into its most dependent part. The anvil is then introduced into the anal stump and the trocar advanced through the transverse stapled line into the pelvis. This is then engaged by the head, and the instrument is closed, bringing the ileal reservoir down to the anal stump. The instrument is fired, and the anastomotic line is carefully examined for completeness.

Hand-sewn

In the case of a hand-sewn anastomosis, the reservoir is constructed to leave an aperture at its most dependent part, which conveniently takes two fingers as an appropriate diameter. Two sutures are placed diametrically opposite on each side of the aperture of the reservoir for subsequent delivery through the anal canal.

Before constructing the anastomosis, a mucosectomy is carried out. This serves two functions: first, it removes diseased tissue from the upper anal canal and hence irradicates recurrent disease, and second, it makes the manual anastomosis easier by advancing it more distally.

The mucosectomy is carried out endo-anally by scissor dissection in the submucosal plane (see Figure 8.4). This is facilitated by the injection of saline containing a small amount of adrenaline (1 : 300 000) into the submucosa, with the effect of lifting the mucosa off the internal sphincter and the circular muscle. The mucosa should be removed as a single specimen rather than in several pieces as this minimizes the possibility of leaving small islands behind. The mucosectomy is taken to within about 0.5 cm above the tips of the anal papillae.

At this stage, the sutures placed on each side of the aperture of the pouch are drawn down through the anal canal by the perineal operator, to be delivered through the anus. They are then inserted into the anal canal in the right and left lateral positions and are tied. This brings the pouch down to the level of the ileo-anal anastomosis; further sutures can then be placed endo-anally to complete it (Figure 4.6 and Plate 7). A suction drain left in the pelvis is removed 12–24 hours later.

Ileostomy

Most surgeons will use a loop ileostomy, the arguments for and against this being discussed in a subsequent chapter. Forming an ileostomy has the merit of increased safety should the patient

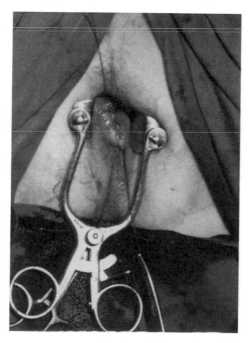

Figure 4.6 Pouch anal anastomosis (see Plate 7).

develop pelvic sepsis from a defect of the ileo-anal anastomosis or pouch. It is common practice to support the loop ileostomy with a rod (Figure 4.7 and Plate 8). The price paid, however, is a second operation to close it, a longer total treatment time and complications related to the stoma.

The disadvantage of not performing a stoma is the severity of sepsis that can occur should the anastomosis leak. This will require an urgent ileostomy in an ill patient and will be necessary in approximately 10 per cent of cases. Patients having a restorative proctocolectomy without a temporary ileostomy should be managed postoperatively with an indwelling catheter in the pouch brought out through the anus.

Postoperative care

Postoperatively, the patient is mobilized and given physiotherapy, stoma and wound care. The drain is removed 12 hours later and the urinary catheter on the fourth or fifth postoperative day. It should be possible to give small amounts of liquid by mouth from the first postoperative day, but the build-up to a full oral intake of liquids and solids will depend on a functioning ileostomy. This usually begins to act on the third or fourth postoperative day. At this time, the rod

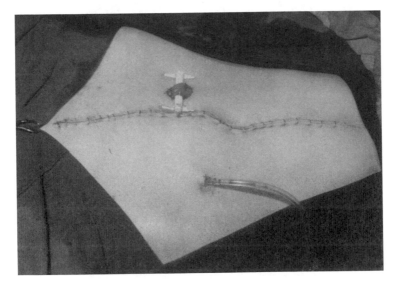

Figure 4.7 Loop ileostomy with rod (see Plate 8).

supporting the loop ileostomy can be removed, which will sometimes improve the action of the stoma.

The stoma should remain pinky red in colour and look healthy in order for it to remain viable. If there is any discolouration in the stoma and it is felt that the bowel is longer viable, inspection by an experienced surgeon, down the stoma using a paediatric sigmoidoscope, will reveal its extent. Careful observation of the stoma is important as revision may be necessary.

Patients should be warned to expect some discharge per anum. This is usually a mixture of altered blood and mucus, and is a normal occurrence in the immediate postoperative period. If the blood is fresh in colour and abundant in volume, an examination under anaesthetic should be considered since this is an indication of sepsis at the anastomosis with secondary haemorrhage.

It is of course important to monitor the vital signs. A raised temperature occurring within the first 24–48 hours is almost always caused by a lung complication. When pyrexia occurs after the fourth day, it is likely to be the result of a wound infection or an intra-abdominal connection. By far the most common site for this is in the pelvis. Digital examination through the anus should be performed to feel for swelling and induration at the ileo-anal anastomotic level. When present, this is usually posterior.

Postoperative complications

This operation has a reputation for a high morbidity, with a reported complication rate of 30 per cent or more in most surgical series. It must be said, however, that the identification of complications and their reporting is a feature of more modern surgical practice and may be a reflection of this rather than of any factor particularly associated with the operation. For example, the complications arising after low anterior resection for carcinoma are similar.

The two most important complications are sepsis and obstruction. When it occurs, sepsis is usually located in the pelvis and is often associated with a degree of breakdown of the ileo-anal anastomosis. An infected haematoma may, however, form in the presence of an intact anastomosis. The incidence of pelvic sepsis is reported to range from 5 to 20 per cent (Dozois et al 1986). The term 'pelvic sepsis' has variable meaning. Some surgeons use it to describe a septic state requiring laparotomy to drain pus or faeces, whereas others use it to indicate any degree of infection within the pelvis, however limited this may be. Despite these semantic difficulties, an average figure for pelvic sepsis of clinical importance requiring drainage (usually endo-anally) is between 5 and 10 per cent.

Pelvic sepsis should be suspected in a patient developing a temperature after a few days. The chest and abdomen should be examined and urine sent for culture. The wound should be carefully examined. Digital examination per anum may reveal its presence. A defect in the anastomosis may also be felt. It is helpful to have an abdominal ultrasound to identify possible foci of infection in the abdomen. Ultrasound is poor at identifying pelvic sepsis since the pouch itself produces confusing images. When initial examination is negative, a computed tomography (CT) scan should be performed. This is much more reliable than ultrasound in identifying pelvic sepsis. An examination under anaesthetic should be carried out to identify and drain any abscess. The occurrence of pelvic sepsis increases the chance of subsequent failure of the operation. At St Mark's Hospital, about one-third of the 10 per cent of patients developing pelvic sepsis ultimately lose the reservoir, giving an overall figure of early failure due to sepsis of 3.3 per cent.

In the early days, obstruction was cited as being a common event, but obstruction requiring surgery to relieve it is now infrequent. It may be that, with the development of parenteral nutrition, surgeons feel able to wait longer for the spontaneous resolution of an obstructive syndrome when it occurs. Episodes are indeed fairly common but usually resolve spontaneously. The cause of obstruction is variable, including a single adhesion, a general matting together of the loops of small bowel by adhesions, torsion and narrowing of the loop stoma.

Haemorrhage may be reactionary or secondary. Reactionary haemorrhage occurring within the first 6 hours following surgery is usually caused by bleeding from a vessel in the pelvis. If the bleeding is significant, the patient will require re-operation. On opening the abdomen, free blood should be cleared and the site of bleeding looked for. This is most likely to be one of three possible locations: the pre-sacral area, the lateral ligaments and the anal stump in cases having a manual anastomosis. It may not be possible to identify and secure the bleeding owing to the presence of the pouch, and it may be necessary to detach the ileo-anal anastomosis to achieve this. The anastomosis can then be immediately remade.

Secondary haemorrhage from the reservoir is indicative of sepsis and usually occurs at 1 week or more. It is indicated by bright blood issuing per anum. An examination under anaesthetic, with facilities to irrigate the pouch and diathermy coagulation, is necessary.

Stoma complications are of two main types: the first includes water and electrolyte depletion, and the second some local problem associated with the stoma itself.

Water and electrolyte depletion is common in the early postoperative period. It is anticipated because the ileum has been defunctioned in order to allow the pouch and anal anastomoses to heal, thus leaving the patient with approximately 30–50 cm of small bowel not functioning. It is not uncommon for patients to experience an output of 2–4 litres in a 24 hour period. This may be due to the stoma being placed too proximally, but in most cases a functional cause is presumed. The output usually settles within days or up to a week or two.

Water and sodium loss is a common problem, and it is important that the ileostomy output is measured and the general condition of the patient monitored to anticipate features of sodium depletion. The symptoms of this include weakness, postural hypotension, anorexia, nausea, tachycardia associated with peripheral vasoconstriction, raised urea and electrolyte levels, low urinary output and acidosis (which will, if severe, lead to renal failure). Whilst the patient is in hospital, it is important to maintain an accurate record of fluid balance. In addition to this, an accurate measurement of whether the patient is sodium depleted can be made by taking a random urine sodium test. The concentration of sodium within the urine should be greater than 20 mmol/l of urine.

The patient may need to use an appliance appropriate for the high output, that is, a urostomy appliance with continuous drainage (Figure 4.8). This not only allows the patient to rest, but also prevents the appliance from over-filling and potentially leaking. Prior to going home, the patient must be made aware of the signs and symptoms of fluid imbalance (Table 4.2).

The possibility of sodium depletion should be explained to all patients at the time of discharge from hospital, and if there is any doubt over the patient's competence to add salt to food, a rehydration

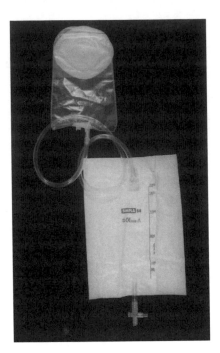

Figure 4.8 High-output system.

Table 4.2 Signs and symptoms of electrolyte imbalance

- Dry mouth and mucous membranes
- Decreased urine output and increased urinary concentration
- Nausea and vomiting
- Sunken (panda) eyes
- Extreme weakness
- Muscle cramps (abdomen or limbs)
- Lethargy
- Tingling or cramping in the feet and hands
- Confusion

solution should be prescribed. Treatment is by sodium replenishment, which may need to be intravenous. The patient should be given an electrolyte mixture and encouraged to add salt to food. Electrolyte mixtures contain sodium in a concentration of about 60 mmol/l, so the patient must understand that two volumes of electrolyte mixture are equivalent in sodium for every one volume of ileostomy effluent lost.

The loop ileostomy

The temporary loop ileostomy serves the purpose of diverting effluent from the anastomotic suture lines, thus aiding the healing of the
reservoir. In practical terms, the temporary loop ileostomy can be
difficult for patients to manage. This is generally because of the
increased likelihood of stomal retraction and mucosal separation,
the corrosive nature of the effluent, resulting from its high content of
prolytic enzymes, a high stomal output leading to water and electrolyte imbalance, and mucosal discharge from the distal end of the
stoma (Figure 4.9 and Plate 9).

These problems are likely to occur within the immediate postoperative period and may prolong the patient's stay in hospital. It is
therefore particularly important for the nurse specialist in stoma care
to be vigilant in order to decrease management problems and to
promote comprehensive rehabilitation. These problems are
discussed in more detail in Chapter 8.

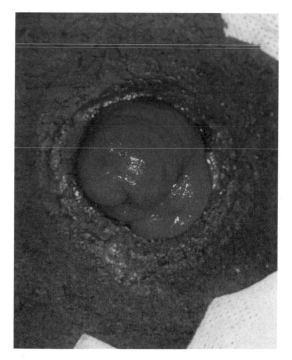

Figure 4.9 Loop ileostomy (see Plate 9).

Closure of the temporary ileostomy

Closing the ileostomy is a relatively minor procedure. In most cases, closure of the ileostomy can be undertaken locally, but there is a 1 per cent risk of laparotomy in order to close the stoma. Normally, an incision is made around the ileostomy in order to release the bowel, the bowel then being closed. Bowel function through the anus usually starts within 12–48 hours after the closure of the temporary ileostomy, and the patient can usually go home within 7 days of the operation.

Function

The patient's function becomes apparent only after the closure of the defunctioning ileostomy. Function in the early post-closure period may be disturbed (although often it is not), and patients should know that it may take weeks or months for frequency to settle and some soiling to resolve. Documentation of function was reported from many surgical units in the early experience of the operation, and this is summarised in the literature (Dozois et al 1986).

Frequency of defaecation ranges from 2 or 3 to over 10 times per 24 hours. This depends to some extent on the type of reservoir used, but, in addition, the pouch transit time should be noted. An important factor influencing pouch function is the total daily volume of ileal effluent. This has been shown to be directly proportional to the daily individual dietary preferences and the absolute volume of the food ingested (Levitt & Kuan 1998).

The most important symptomatic improvement following restorative proctocolectomy for those with ulcerative colitis is the absence of urgency, which has been reported to occur in around only 5 per cent of patients (Naysmith et al 1986). It is relief from this that the colitic patient appreciates most. A certain frequency appears to be well tolerated provided that it is possible to postpone defaecation by 30–60 minutes, which the majority of patients can do. This beneficial aspect of the operation has not received sufficient attention. Frequency itself may be related to various factors, for example the frequency of micturition, periods of introspection, the fear of passing stool rather than flatus and so on. For patients with FAP, an adaptation to the frequency of pouch function needs to take place as the presenting symptoms are in no way as extreme as they are in the patient with ulcerative colitis.

Continence is normal in 60–80 per cent of patients. Faecal incontinence is uncommon, occurring in less than 5 per cent of patients, but some night-soiling and mucous discharge occurs in about 10–20 per cent of cases (Kohler et al 1992).

Pouch evacuation

Defaecation in those with a colon and rectum is a complex process involving propulsive colonic contractions, coordinated pelvic floor relaxation and raised intra-abdominal pressure (Groom et al 1994). In pouch patients, the pouch fills progressively once any foods or liquids have been consumed. There is a steady rise in baseline pouch pressure and the occurrence of pouch contraction waves of increasing frequency and amplitude, patients experiencing an increasing urge to defaecate. Pouch contraction waves do not, however, appear to be propulsive in nature, and evacuation is achieved in the normal manner combined with relaxation of the pelvic floor and external anal sphincter (Levitt & Kuan 1998). Pouch patients not experiencing any symptomatic difficulties emptying their pouch are generally able to evacuate almost 100 per cent of their pouch contents (Levitt et al 1991).

Pouch absorption

Although malabsorption syndromes are rarely seen after pouch formation, subtle but significant abnormalities do occur. The preservation of a normal terminal ileal absorptive surface seems to allow pouch patients to retain their ability to absorb substances, including both primary bile acids and unbound vitamin B12–intrinsic factor complexes (Gadacz et al 1997). It would, however, appear to be the bacterial overgrowth within the pouch that causes problems (Levitt & Kuan 1998). At St Mark's Hospital, it is common practice to take annual blood tests for full blood count, urea and electrolytes, and folate level, 5 years post-pouch formation in order to monitor any significant malabsorption.

Perianal skin care

Frequency and leakage when present, will lead to anal soreness, and it should be stressed to patients that they should take great care of

their perianal skin. An explanation of why soreness might occur
helps them to understand the importance of good perianal skin care
(Table 4.3). A good barrier cream should be recommended, such as
one with a zinc oxide or aluminium base. At St Mark's Hospital,
patients are offered a 'bum-bag'; this allows them to experiment with
'lotions and potions' to see which is appropriate for their individual
need (Figure 4.10).

Patients more often than not describe a rectal burning and/or anal
itch as being more troublesome than perianal skin soreness. It is
thought that this arises from irritation from effluent at the pouch–anal

Table 4.3 Tips for good perianal skin care

- Keep the area clean by washing (not too vigorously) and drying after every bowel motion
- Avoid rubbing with a soapy rough flannel
- Use moist toilet paper (available at chemists and supermarkets), preferably one with a very low alcohol content or none at all
- Keep the anal area dry
- Avoid perfumed talcum powder
- Wear cotton underwear and avoid close-fitting trousers or tights
- Avoid an excessive use of ointments and creams, and ensure that these are completely washed away prior to re-application
- Consider thickening the bowel motions by changing the diet and/or taking anti-diarrhoeal drugs such as Imodium or codeine phosphate
- If the problem persists, seek medical attention

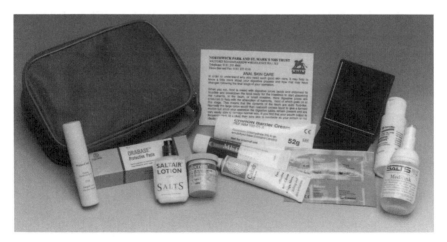

Figure 4.10 A 'bum-bag'.

anastomosis. A haemorrhoid preparation and/or aloe vera gel (80 per cent or more pure) can be helpful in this instance. Confirmation that a fissure is not present must, however, also be established. A fissure is a 'crack-like' lesion of the skin and is commonly found in the anal canal. It can be treated topically with either a steroid-based cream or glyceryl trinitrate ointment, however, the latter can lead to varying degrees of incontinence during treatment.

Drugs

Many patients are reliant upon the anti-motility drugs such as loperamide hydrochloride (Imodium), codeine phosphate and co-phenotrope (Lomotil) in the initial stages of their pouch functioning. Caution must be applied in not over-prescribing these drugs, with the attendant risk of obstruction. After a time, however, patients are able to titrate the dose in order to achieve a satisfactory pouch function. Most pouch patients are able to wean themselves off these medications 2 years post-pouch formation.

Loperamide is the anti-motility drug of choice as its side-effects are minimal; it is considered safe to administer during pregnancy. It is of interest to note that Imodium elixir has a higher concentration of glucose, and can therefore, if taken in large doses, can cause frequency of pouch function. Most pouch patients administer Imodium in tablet or capsule form.

Long-term complications

Long-term, patients may develop anaemia, so haemoglobin levels should be checked regularly. In some cases, the anaemia may arise from vitamin B12 deficiency, but it is more often associated with a low serum iron level. Long-term septic complications in the form of a pouch–vaginal or pouch–perineal fistula can occur. Poor function may never resolve, and mucosal inflammation of the pouch may occur.

Thus failure, defined as a need to remove the reservoir or establish an ileostomy for an indefinite period of time, occurs throughout the period of follow-up. Over a 10 year period at St Mark's Hospital, the failure rate in the first year was 7 per cent, rising by 10 years to almost 15 per cent. There is therefore a steady failure rate over a long period of time, although patients can be reassured that if all is well at 1 year, the failure rate falls to less than 10 per cent.

The most common cause of failure in the immediate postoperative period is sepsis, other reasons such as ischaemia of the reservoir being very uncommon. In the long term, failure mainly results from three causes: chronic sepsis, usually manifesting as fistulation from the ileo-anal anastomosis, poor function and pouchitis.

Pouch fistula

A fistula is an abnormal opening (hole) from one cavity tracking through to another. Infection around the join between the pouch and the anus can sometimes track its way out to the exterior. In females, this usually manifests itself as a pouch–vaginal fistula, whereas in males, infection penetrates through the buttock wall. Whatever the route, the effect is for faeces to leak out, causing incontinence. Managing the condition can be difficult. Most surgeons recommend further surgery to correct the defect and/or form a temporary loop ileostomy in order to allow a rest period, with the hope that the fistula will heal. Should the fistula fail to heal, the patient will be advised to consider the removal of the pouch.

Poor function

Some patients experience difficulty in emptying their pouch, so much so that they feel they have not completely emptied it but need to return to the toilet to achieve this. From the literature, the true incidence of evacuation disorders is unclear (Levitt & Kuan 1998). In a recent survey (Bond et al 1997) investigating quality of life issues, half of the respondents expressed difficulty in evacuating their pouch. Of those who experienced difficulty, 5 per cent used a catheter to aid evacuation, and a further 5 per cent had to irrigate their pouch.

The reasons for poor function may include stricture and/or angulation of the pouch–anal anastomosis (Levitt & Kuan 1998) as well as retained rectal mucosa (see Chapter 8). Other causes, such as mechanical problems, are not completely understood. In either case, investigations, for example a defaecating pouchogram, anal physiology and pouch compliance, will assist the decision to determine how best to treat the problem. The defaecating pouchogram will illustrate how the pouch is functioning, that is, whether or not there is a total completion of emptying, whilst anal physiology will detect any defect within the anal canal, and pouch compliance will demonstrate overall pouch function. In general, those patients with higher compliance values have better function with fewer pouch evacuations per day and less leakage.

Spontaneous defaecation may occasionally not occur. If there is difficulty in evacuating the pouch, patients may need to pay particular attention to their posture while defaecating. When on the toilet, they should ensure that they are relaxed and seated in an upright position with their feet slightly raised, for example with the aid of a telephone directory or waste paper basket. This will encourage the use of the abdominal oblique muscles, which are essential for complete defaecation, rather than straining and pushing through the perineum. In the latter, patients are likely to be contracting their anal sphincter muscles rather than relaxing them in order to aid defaecation.

Although it is uncommon, patients may be taught to insert a medina catheter (see Figure 5.3) into the pouch in order to aid evacuation. Consideration may also be given to the use of biofeedback treatment, in which patients are re-taught how to evacuate their pouch using the appropriate abdominal muscles. On occasion, surgical intervention is required. Many pouch patients with an 'S'-configurated pouch use the medina catheter to aid evacuation.

Pouchitis

Despite all that has been written on pouchitis, the published literature indicates that it is only rarely a cause of failure, accounting for about 3 per cent of the total pouch population (Pemberton et al 1987, Lohmuller et al 1990). Little is known about the aetiology of pouchitis. Risk factors include the presence of extra-intestinal manifestations, primary sclerosing cholangitis, the cessation of smoking and the previous course of the disease (Kuhbacher et al 1998).

In some patients, the mucosa develops acute inflammatory changes associated with symptoms. The changes can be seen endoscopically and must be present microscopically to make the diagnosis. Pouchitis requires histological confirmation to make the diagnosis, just as proctitis does (Shepherd 1989). There is no justification for diagnosing pouchitis on the basis of symptoms such as frequency since there are other causes for this, as discussed in Chapter 8.

All patients undergoing restorative proctocolectomy, whether for ulcerative colitis or FAP, demonstrate a degree of villous atrophy within the small bowel mucosa of the reservoir (Scott & Phillips 1989). Some patients with ulcerative colitis in addition develop an inflammatory response. This does not seem to happen in FAP, and pouchitis probably does not occur in this disease; more recently, however, adenomas have been identified through flexible pouchoscopy. It should be noted that pouchitis does not occur while the pouch is defunctioned. It is recognized that patients described similar symptoms, but this is not pouchitis in the true sense of the word.

There is every indication that the mucosal changes begin early after the closure of the ileostomy. By 3 months, three groups of patients seem to have emerged (Setti-Carraro et al 1994), these remaining true to type over the years. The first group (50 per cent) includes patients who never develop acute inflammatory changes or episodes of pouchitis. In the second group (40 per cent), episodes of histological inflammation associated with symptoms occur that settle either on treatment or spontaneously. These may recur at varying intervals, sometimes very prolonged ones. The third group (10 per cent) includes patients who, from within a few weeks of closure of the ileostomy, develop chronic unremitting inflammation of the reservoir associated with symptoms. It is this group which presents a chronic clinical problem, possibly requiring the subsequent excision of the reservoir.

The cause of pouchitis is not known, but the fact that it occurs in colitic patients must be significant. Current research is attempting to define the nature of the inflammatory response, including the cytokine profile and the timing and evolution of the inflammatory changes. It is quite likely, given the response to antibiotics, that intraluminal bacteria play a major role. It should be appreciated that the bacterial concentration within the small bowel reservoir rises to over a million times that of the normal terminal ileum.

Despite much empiricism, the only effective treatment for pouchitis is antibiotics, including metronidazole, ciprofloxacin and Augmentin, although these may not work in patients with chronic unremitting pouchitis. Anti-inflammatory treatment with steroids, 5-aminosalicylic acid derivatives and immunosuppression does not seem to help patients with pouchitis. Some surgeons choose to form a loop ileostomy in order to rest the pouch in the hope that the inflammation will settle.

Cuffitis

Cuffitis is a cause of pouch dysfunction after double-stapled restorative proctocolectomy (Thompson-Fawcett et al 1999). It is defined as inflammation at the columnar cuff and is situated above the anal transitional zone. In a study of 113 patients, 13 per cent were found to have acute inflammation that ultimately needed treatment.

Quality of life

Pouch patients have been asked about their quality of life after a restorative operation compared with life with an ileostomy (Salter 1992a, Bond et al 1997). It must be appreciated that these patients had a strong desire to avoid a permanent ileostomy so they might therefore be prejudiced towards feeling that the pouch operation had been worthwhile. Nevertheless, all had experienced an ileostomy at some stage during their treatment. The results of such surveys have shown that about 80 per cent of patients who have not had to have a subsequent permanent ileostomy think that their quality of life is better after pouch surgery than it was when they had a temporary loop ileostomy. This decision is on the basis of such aspects as body image, clothing, sport, work and sex appeal.

Patients' expectations of pouch surgery remain high. There is often an expression of hope that the ileo-anal pouch will ultimately bring about a return to an acceptable degree of normality, that is, disease-free and with control of bowel function – life without a permanent ileostomy (Williams 1998).

As illustrated earlier, pouch function is unpredictable in that, although urgency and blood in the stools have been eliminated, it is uncertain how many times the pouch will function. Many patients curtail their lifestyle, for example restricting their diet or changing their meal patterns as well as reducing their social activities to what they become 'comfortable with', in order to maintain everyday living. Patients need to be informed that this may prove to be the case for them too.

It is well documented that giving patients information prior to impending surgery can reduce their emotional response and facilitate coping, thus aiding recovery (Salter 1988). Williams (1998), in a study reflecting patients' expectations of pouch surgery, noted that it is important for nurses at the preoperative consultation to clarify patients' expectations and identify their hopes through active listening, giving support and guidance with the aim of focusing the patient on a more realistic outlook of life with a pouch. This will in turn help new pouch patients to develop coping strategies postoperatively, thus adapting to their new lifestyle with greater ease.

CHAPTER 5

The Kock pouch and nursing care

Julia Williams and Peter Hawley

During the twentieth century, there has been much progress in patient management following proctocolectomy. Surgery has advanced from the ileum protruding through the abdominal wall as an ileostomy to the ileum being reconstructed into a reservoir as an internal pouch. It is widely acknowledged that the psychological trauma for patients with newly formed stomas is enormous (Devlin et al 1971, Bond et al 1997), and therefore the adaptation process is often prolonged (Price 1990). In the early years of surgical development, many ileostomy patients suffered with intestinal obstruction and peristomal skin soreness. Although they remained 'disease-free', they also remained unhappy with the continual wearing of an appliance, concerned about their daily physiological constraints and unhappy with their body change, struggling to seek a new lifestyle. Obviously, over time not only has surgical management changed dramatically, but so too has the technology beind manufacturing appliances, thus making adaptation for the patient easier.

It was in the late 1960s that Professor Nils Kock created the idea of a surgical procedure that would provide storage capacity as well as restore control over the discharge of waste from the body. He believed that if an intestinal reservoir could be created by a technique similar to that used to collect urine following total cystectomy, patients could gain more control of their lives. This new anatomical arrangement consisted of a nipple valve and a pouch that resided within the abdominal cavity, eliminating the need to wear a bag (Spencer & Barnett 1982). Although the Kock pouch (or continent ileostomy) procedure is not now deemed to be the first surgical choice for a patient with ulcerative colitis or familial adenomatous polyposis (FAP), and is therefore not performed very often, it is important to highlight the procedure, the nursing care of these patients and the implications for patients with regard to their lifestyle.

Patient selection

The majority of patients who undergo the Kock pouch procedure will be those with ulcerative colitis or FAP, although the first choice of surgical management for these are a colectomy and ileorectal anastomosis (IRA) or restorative proctocolectomy (RPC) respectively. There may, however, be some instances, identified through patient assessment, in which it is noted that the anal sphincter is weak or indeed the rectum and anus are so diseased that it is not possible to preserve the anal sphincter. This would render the patient incontinent of faeces should he or she undergo either IRA or RPC, so the Kock pouch should be considered for such circumstances.

Some controversy surrounds whether the patient with Crohn's disease should be offered a Kock pouch. Early literature (Handelsman et al 1993) suggests that the Kock pouch is contraindicated in Crohn's disease, highlighting a risk of complications such as fistula and leakage. Most patients with Crohn's disease who have had a Kock pouch are those in whom the diagnosis was not known at the time of the original operation. The pouch was therefore constructed in the belief that the underlying disease was ulcerative colitis, the eventual diagnosis of Crohn's disease being revealed by histological examination of the colectomy specimen or as a result of complications necessitating the removal of the pouch.

Some studies suggest that those with colonic Crohn's disease and a normal small bowel can be offered a Kock pouch as an alternative to permanent ileostomy as long as they are made aware of the possible implications. Morbidity rates no different from the rate of complications in patients with ulcerative colitis or FAP have been reported (Gerber et al 1983). It is unwise to construct a Kock pouch at the time of emergency surgery for colitis and/or in those receiving high-dose, long-term steroid therapy (Keighley & Williams 1993).

The current rationale for offering a Kock pouch is somewhat different from that advocated by Kock in 1969. At that time, the

Kock pouch was the only alternative to a conventional ileostomy in patients with severe rectal disease. Nowadays, the operation is considered only when the ileo-anal reservoir has failed as a result of poor function or in patients who have in the past had a procto-colectomy with end-ileostomy. Despite the recognized higher re-operation rate, it is felt that the Kock pouch procedure has a place for those patients who are highly motivated and wish to avoid wearing a permanent ileostomy bag. The indications for a Kock pouch may currently be more extensive since this is viewed as an alternative to a conventional stoma for patients with congenital anorectal anomalies, faecal incontinence and multiple colorectal carcinoma.

Most patients opt for a Kock pouch out of a desire to avoid wearing a permanent bag, for sexual, social and sometimes religious reasons. It is of the utmost importance that the patient is psychologically stable and able to grasp the concept of the Kock pouch. A lack of understanding or not having a full appreciation of the procedure, in addition to poor social circumstances, may lead to difficulties in coping with the pouch as patients will need to learn how to intubate and irrigate the pouch whilst maintaining a reasonable level of hygiene.

The surgical procedure

The aim of surgery is to achieve a pouch with a capacity of between 800 and 1000 ml that is completely continent of gas and faeces, and can be emptied by the passage of a catheter no more than three or four times a day, without the patient needing to wake at night in order to drain it. The stoma should be invisible under any clothing. There should be minimal mucous discharge, and complete control should be achieved merely by the application of a disposable dressing over the stoma. Intubation of the pouch should take no more than 20 minutes and there should be no difficulties or complications whilst intubating the pouch. There should also be no limitations on sporting activities, work opportunities, sexual activity, travel or social functioning.

Preoperative phase

It is advisable prior to surgery to select a site on the abdominal wall for the location of the continent ileostomy. The stoma should be located 2–4 cm above the pubic hairline. In contrast to the conventional ileostomy, the stoma may reside in close proximity to bony prominences or skin surface irregularities since an appliance is not necessary in the long term; it is, however, still advisable to site the stoma within the rectus sheath. If the patient already has an ileostomy, it may be difficult to site the Kock pouch, as the optimal position is likely to be beneath the appliance.

Preoperative teaching includes providing information on preoperative care and issues unique to Kock pouch management. Patients will need to be extremely well informed on the implications of the surgery prior to coming into hospital. Little patient information literature is available, so it is important that the patient not only gains information from an experienced clinical nurse specialist in stoma care, but also has the opportunity to speak with other people who have undergone this procedure. Patients should be allowed to discuss their anxieties and concerns, during which the nurse specialist will be able to assess the patients' suitability to undergo such a procedure. Patients may also wish to familiarize themselves with the equipment needed to care for the Kock pouch, for example the medina catheter, the bladder syringe and the stoma cap (Hampton & Bryant 1992).

Although the procedure may vary slightly as a result of the surgeon's preference and technique, the basic principles underlying Kock pouch construction are constant. Once the colectomy has taken place, the ileum is mobilized in preparation for the construction of the reservoir. The pouch is made from the distal 45 cm of ileum. Two 15 cm loops of adjacent ileum are sewn together and then folded into a 'U' shape in order create the reservoir. This section of bowel is then folded horizontally, and the apex is brought to the opening of the proximal limb and sutured in place, creating opposing peristaltic forces within the pouch. The left or efferent outflow loop is closed. For ease of construction, the inflow or afferent loop of the pouch is sutured after the valve has been completed.

To create the valve, the distal 15 cm of ileum is intussuscepted into the pouch. The nipple is then secured inside the pouch using a staple gun. Additional rows of staples are placed on the inverted bowel in order to secure the nipple valve. Other pouch configurations, such as a two-loop 'J', can be used to construct the reservoir.

Pouch continence is checked by placing a non-crushing clamp on the bowel proximal to the pouch and inserting a medina catheter through the nipple valve. Air is injected, and the suture lines are checked for leakage. If all is intact, the air is removed and the stoma completed. A small opening is made in the peritoneum just large enough to allow the distal ileum to pass through. The efferent limb of the pouch is then passed through the abdominal wall layers to the skin, where it is attached by suturing the stoma flush with the skin (see Figure 5.1).

A medina catheter is inserted through the nipple valve into the reservoir and sutured in place to the surface of the skin. The medina

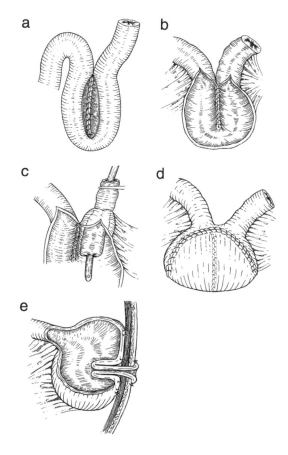

Figure 5.1 Construction of a Kock pouch.

catheter is then connected to a closed drainage system. A 'beehive dressing' is used to secure and support the catheter. The beehive dressing will also prevent the medina catheter from kinking, thus maintaining its patency and allowing free drainage of the pouch.

Postoperative phase

The postoperative management of a patient with a Kock pouch may vary slightly depending on the surgeon's preference. The nursing care plan (Table 5.1) should, however, also include the usual nursing measures utilized following extensive abdominal and perineal surgery, such as vital sign observations, fluid monitoring and wound care. The continent ileostomy stoma should be observed to ensure viability. Any signs of bleeding from the pouch should be thoroughly investigated and the surgeon notified immediately.

Most patients will remain nil by mouth for 3–4 days until the bowel begins to function. When this occurs, patients can begin to take sips of water (or ice), building slowly towards free fluids and then to a low-residue diet. Dietary supplements may be required. The medina catheter drainage system must be observed to ensure free drainage of the newly formed pouch (Figure 5.2, p. 106). It is important during the early stages of the healing process that the pouch is not placed under any tension. Once the patient begins to eat, the risk of blockage of the medina catheter increases. It may be necessary to flush the catheter with 20–30 ml of normal saline twice a day until it is evident that it is free-flowing. For this reason too the medina catheter will remain in place for 4–6 weeks.

It is likely that the patient will find it difficult to care for the medina catheter drainage system and beehive dressing for a long period of time, the management of the catheter being eased by the use of a stoma appliance (Figure 5.3, p. 106). On the fifth postoperative day, the suture securing the medina catheter to the surface of the skin should be slipped and trimmed but not removed from the medina catheter itself. The suture should remain wrapped around the catheter in order to act as a guideline for patients to ensure that the catheter remains in the pouch at all times. This suture line is also helpful during the patient's learning process. Once this suture has been slipped, the catheter's main anchorage is the clip at the end of the drainage appliance.

Most patients have experienced caring for a stoma so the practicalities of stoma care are usually re-established with ease. When

Table 5.1: Nursing care plan for the postoperative care unique to a patient with a Kock pouch

Problem	Expected outcome	Nursing intervention
1. Care of the medina catheter drainage system	To ensure free drainage of the newly formed Kock pouch	a. The medina catheter will remain in position within the Kock pouch for 4–6 weeks b. The nurse will ensure that the pouch contents are draining properly so that the pouch does not become full or block c. The catheter will remain on continuous drainage. The nurse will teach the patient to 'milk' the tubing if necessary d. Five days postoperatively, the nurse will gently flush the catheter with 20–30 ml of normal saline e. The drainage system will be renewed daily f. Fluid balance will be monitored
2. Care and renewal of beehive dressing	To support the medina catheter and maintain peristomal skin integrity	a. The patient will feel comfortable and confident to mobilize with the catheter supported in position b. The nurse will ensure that the dressing supports the catheter well in order to allow pouch drainage and to keep the catheter in place c. The dressing will be renewed as necessary to ensure that the tubing remains in the pouch and does not become bent or kinked d. Five days postoperatively, the suture should be slipped yet remain wrapped around the catheter as a guideline e. The patient should be re-educated about basic stoma care
3. Intubation of the Kock pouch	For the patient to be confident to intubate the pouch and defaecate as necessary	a. Preoperatively, the nurse will familiarize the patient with the medina catheter, bladder syringe and stoma cap b. 4–6 weeks postoperatively, using a teaching programme, the nurse will show the patient how to intubate the pouch, using the catheter and lubricating gel, by demonstration and then by participation c. The nurse will teach the patient to empty the pouch 3–4 hourly initially d. The nurse will educate the patient regarding diet and fluid intake e. The nurse will demonstrate the irrigation technique to the patient f. Patients with a Kock pouch should be encouraged to carry with them information regarding the pouch and appropriate contact numbers

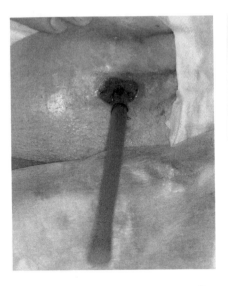

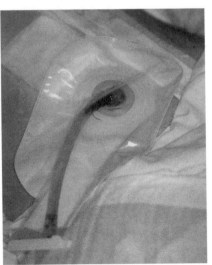

Figure 5.2 (On the left) The medina catheter in situ (see Plate 10).

Figure 5.3 (On the right) Medina in pouch with stoma appliance (see Plate 11).

choosing an appliance, the preference is for a two-piece system so that skin integrity is maintained. If the patient is more familiar with a one-piece system, this can be adapted by using a washer at the skin surface, thus maintaining skin integrity. Patients will need additional instruction in cleaning the catheter whilst renewing the appliance.

Once the patient is maintaining a soft diet, the risk of blockage of the catheter from a food bolus increases. If this were to occur, the patient would complain of abdominal discomfort and distension, and describe the absence of motion into the stoma appliance. It is important that the pouch is not put under any tension during the 4–6 week healing period so the patient will need to be taught how to irrigate (flush) the pouch prior to discharge (Table 5.2).

During irrigation, the nurse should examine the stoma for viability and check the peristomal skin for integrity. If fluid should bypass the medina catheter and seep around the stoma during the procedure, it may indicate that the catheter is in the valve rather than the pouch. The patient may need to be taught how to re-introduce the medina catheter gently into the pouch. Once irrigation has been completed and it is noted that the output from the pouch is less than anticipated, the medina catheter should be removed to examine its

Table 5.2 Continent ileostomy irrigation

Equipment needed
A bladder syringe
Tap water (500ml–1l)
A container to hold the water
Equipment for draining the catheter

Procedure
1. Wash your hands
2. Lubricate the catheter, and drain the pouch in the usual manner
3. Leave the catheter in place when you have finished
4. Fill the bladder syringe with 30–50 ml of water (or enough for the syringe to be handled)
5. Insert the syringe into the free end of the catheter
6. Gently but firmly push the water into the pouch
7. Remove the syringe from the catheter and allow the water to flow freely via the catheter
8. Repeat until the fluid comes back clear

NB: Do not instill more fluid if the initial fluid does not return. In this case, use different techniques to aid emptying, for example coughing, standing and sitting, and gently moving the catheter in and out of the pouch.

eyelets for blockage or kinking of the tube. A new catheter can be inserted in either case. This should be carried out under the guidance of the clinical nurse specialist in stoma care or the consultant surgeon. Patients are often worried that the medina catheter will fall out of the pouch. They should be reassured that although this should not happen, because of the positioning of the clip and the capacity of the stoma appliance, if it were to occur the medina catheter can simply be re-inserted.

Complications

Early complications

The principal early complications during the patient's initial hospital stay are those associated with any major laparotomy. If the operation is being performed as a primary procedure at the time of procto-colectomy, complications such as delayed perineal wound healing and pelvic abscess may develop. If, however, the operation is being performed in a patient with an established stoma, there may be complications as a result of previous adhesions. The main early complications will include necrosis of the nipple valve, parastomal fistula, paralytic ileus, intestinal obstruction and perineal abscess.

The blood supply to the pouch only rarely become compromised, leading to necrosis. Nipple valve necrosis does not necessarily result in faecal peritonitis or fistula since the valve may de-slough, leaving healthy intact mucosa. Nipple valve ischaemia, however, requires surgical intervention to reconstruct the valve. Pouch excision and the formation of an end-ileostomy are not common in this instance. Localized ischaemia may result in a nipple valve fistula, which may not become evident until the catheter is removed.

The pouch itself may leak intestinal contents as a result of suture line dehiscence, catheter damage or an area of ischaemia between the nipple valve and the pouch closure line, leading to faecal peritonitis. In each case, removal is not necessary but proximal diversion, i.e. loop jejunostomy, is advisable.

Late complications

Long-term complications associated with the Kock pouch include a sliding nipple valve, a pouch/enterocutaneous fistula, stenosis of the nipple valve, difficult intubation, prolapse of the pouch, pouchitis, recurrent Crohn's disease and obstruction. Overall, most Kock pouch complications are treated conservatively (Keighley & Williams 1993), and most surgeons will endeavour to preserve the pouch provided the patient's life is not threatened in any way.

At least 20 per cent of all complications with the Kock pouch are associated with nipple valve dysfunction (Ecker et al 1996). The intussuscepted portion of the bowel slides upon itself, and the integrity of the nipple valve is lost. This will make it difficult or impossible to pass the catheter into the pouch. The patient is likely to complain of slight oozing to severe incontinence of faeces. A stoma plug may be helpful if the oozing is minimal, but surgical reconstruction of the nipple valve may be necessary. Some patients experience excessive mucous discharge, which can be caused by pouchitis, unrecognized Crohn's disease or an elongated efferent limb.

A fistula can occur in the nipple valve and/or within the pouch, i.e. an enterocutaneous fistula. Incontinence is evident from either the stoma site or the midline incision. It can be treated conservatively by inserting a medina catheter into the pouch, thus requiring the patient to wear a stoma appliance. In both instances, skin integrity must be maintained. Surgical diversion may be necessary only if the fistula does not heal. Rarely does the pouch have to be removed. Even with acute problems, whether from the original surgery or from other acute abdominal situations, such as trauma or peritonitis, all the alternatives should be evaluated carefully before excising the pouch. A loop jejunostomy might be considered to allow time for proper evaluation. The pouch can then, if indicated, be removed later on an elective basis. Recurrent Crohn's disease is one of a few indications for pouch removal.

Some surgeons believe that the Barnett continent intestinal reservoir, a modification of the original Kock pouch, reduces the incidence of valve slippage and fistula formation (Mullen et al 1995). This procedure has been performed since 1988 and modifies the valve and design of the pouch. Mullen et al (1995) studied 510 cases in which patients received a Barnett continent intestinal reservoir instead of Kock pouch. The study highlighted a 92 per cent satisfaction rate with pouch function, with a re-operation rate of 12 per cent for those with major complications, revealing a significant improvement in general quality of life, state of mind and overall health.

Stenosis of the nipple valve may occur following fistula formation (within the valve) or other scarring, dilatation then being necessary in order to correct the narrowed passage way. This has proved to be extremely troublesome (Gottlieb et al. 1991). Another problem is prolapsing of the nipple valve, as it completely defeats the aim of the operation in that the patient is incontinent because of a significant discrepancy in size between the diameter of the outflow tract at the base of the valve, where the pouch meets the abdominal wall, and the diameter of the stoma itself. Stretching of the abdominal wall, such as with overexertion (e.g. heavy lifting) on the part of the patient, weight gain and pregnancy are all contributing factors. Most pouches can be reduced, and the patient can be taught how to do this, but once the wall has weakened, it is probable that the valve will continue to prolapse, and surgical intervention may be required. It is still possible to intubate the pouch, but most patients prefer in addition to wear an appliance because of the excessive leakage.

Many patients complain of difficulty intubating their Kock pouch from time to time. This is generally because they have allowed their pouch to overfill. This in turn distorts the valve and changes the positioning of the pouch, therefore creating resistance when attempting to pass the medina catheter into the pouch. Once several unsuccessful intubation attempts have been made by the patient, the stoma can become oedematous, leading to even greater difficulty, and the patient may begin to panic. In this instance, the patient will need to seek medical support from the local hospital.

Only an experienced clinical nurse specialist in stoma care or a colorectal surgeon should make an attempt at intubating the Kock pouch. If this still proves difficult, an introducer through the centre of the medina catheter will make it slightly more rigid and thus ease the process. The patient will occasionally need endoscopic support to allow successful intubation. Patient education will obviously help to prevent such a situation.

Pouchitis occurs in approximately 10–20 per cent of Kock pouches (De Silva & Mortensen 1992). As with the ileo-anal pouch, it is felt that pouchitis is more predominant in those who suffer with ulcerative colitis or Crohn's disease and does not occur in those with FAP. Although the cause is unknown, it is generally felt that inflammation within the pouch is caused by intestinal stasis with bacterial overgrowth. Symptoms include increased pouch intubation, bleeding and incontinence. Endoscopy and pouch mucosal biopsy provide confirmation of pouchitis. Treatment includes antibiotic therapy with, for example, metronidazole or ciprofloxacin. If the problem persists, a combination of steroids and/or aminosalicylates may be prescribed.

The evidence for malabsorption, bacterial overgrowth and mucosal changes occurring in a Kock pouch is unclear. Some reports (Schjonsby et al 1977, Loeschke et al 1980) have shown significant vitamin B12 malabsorption and steatorrhoea, whereas others (Nilsson et al 1979) show only a marked increase in bacterial overgrowth. Loeschke et al (1980) felt that the mucosal structure was usually normal except for some villus clubbing in a few pouch biopsy samples. They believed that the histological changes were not sufficiently severe to account for any substantial malabsorption.

Patient education

The patient is seen 4–6 weeks after discharge in the outpatient department. Here the medina catheter is removed and the patient is taught how to intubate the pouch. Passing a catheter through a stoma appears to be a fairly straightforward procedure, but to many patients it is a frightening and unnerving experience. The sensation of passing a catheter, albeit not painful, is different from anything the patient has previously experienced. The need for allowing time must be stressed, and reassurance must be given that the patient will learn to care for the Kock pouch.

It is the role of the clinical nurse specialist in stoma care to teach the patient the intubation process and demonstrate the procedure to the patient. Prior to leaving the outpatient department and travelling home, the patient needs to show that he or she has understood how to intubate and irrigate the pouch.

The patient should be informed that the stoma has no nerve endings so intubation will not be painful. The pouch will initially need emptying 3–4 hourly until the patient adapts and the pouch capacity increases. The recognition of when the pouch is full and requires emptying will be determined by abdominal fullness. It is extremely important to provide support and verbal feedback to the patient during this learning process. The interval between intubations gradually increases until the pouch can be intubated only 2–4 times a day.

The teaching process usually begins with the patient sitting up in bed, but he or she must be confident enough to try to intubate in the bathroom, either sitting on the toilet or a bathroom stool, prior to leaving hospital. Some prefer to stand during intubation. The amount of time needed for pouch intubation and drainage will vary from 5 to 20 minutes depending on which foods have been eaten and how much irrigation is required.

The catheter is usually placed in a slightly downward position for insertion during pouch intubation, but this may vary. Resistance caused by the pressure of the pouch contents on the nipple valve may be encountered after the catheter has been inserted about 5–8 cm. The patient should be instructed that anxiety may cause the abdominal muscles to tighten, which can lead to a difficult intubation.

The medina catheter tip is lubricated with a water-soluble lubricant. If the patient takes a deep breath in and applies gentle pressure on the catheter whilst exhaling, it usually slides into the pouch with little difficulty. The patient will modify this intubation technique as he or she gains confidence with the procedure.

If the pouch contents do not drain easily through the medina catheter, several techniques can be employed to help the process along.

The patient may irrigate the pouch with 30–40 ml of tap water at a time, up to a total volume of 500–1000 ml or until the output becomes clear. Above all, he or she should be encouraged to relax. In addition, bearing down on the abdominal muscles as if forcing a bowel movement, whilst gently massaging the abdomen, can help. The catheter may also be slowly moved in and out of the pouch. Some patients change their position from sitting to standing, or give a cough, in order to assist with drainage. Again, each individual patient will learn to adapt to the ways in which his or her own Kock pouch will empty.

When the pouch feels empty, the medina catheter should be gently and slowly removed to prevent damage to the pouch, nipple valve or stoma. Folding or pinching the end of the catheter during removal will assist in preventing leakage. A small amount of bleeding is not unusual, especially during the early days of the learning process. Some patients use a protective covering under the catheter to prevent soiling, but once confidence has been gained, there is no longer a need for this.

It is important that the equipment goes everywhere with the patient. This will include:

- a medina catheter;
- lubricating gel;
- soft wipes;
- a stoma cap or cover;
- a bladder syringe and bottle for water (only if the patient irrigates regularly).

Individual Kock pouch patients will develop their own routine of care and management. Some irrigate or flush the pouch after each intubation, whereas others flush only once a day, less or not at all. When flushing or irrigating the pouch, some patients recommend using slightly warm water in order to aid the emptying process.

The life of the medina catheter may vary from a few weeks to a few months. It is acknowledged that, when new, the catheter can feel hard and rigid. With regular usage, it softens and is therefore easier to insert into the Kock pouch. Patients tend to keep two or three medina catheters on the go at any one time and are advised to renew them on a monthly basis. Table 5.3 outlines guidelines for the care of medina catheters.

Table 5.3 Guidelines for cleaning and storing medina catheters

- Wash the catheter with soap and water
- Rinse the soap and water through the inside of the catheter
- Rinse the catheter well
- Hang the catheter to drip dry over a clean surface such as a towel
- When the catheter is dry, place it in a clean zip-lock-type plastic bag for storage

As the continent ileostomy is made from the small bowel (ileum), the surface of the stoma will be similar to that of an ileostomy. It is thus likely that there will be a slight mucous discharge from the stoma. Most patients wear stoma caps, some adapting soft absorbent dressings or even a sticking plaster. In some cases, some patients will produce excess mucous, which is faecally stained. The peristomal skin is likely to become excoriated and should be treated as for any peristomal skin soreness using a hydrocolloid base.

Quality of life

Some studies post a patient satisfaction rate as high as 98 per cent despite recurrent problems such as pouchitis and nipple valve dysfunction that require re-operation (Gerber et al 1983). One patient's words sum up the overall feelings towards Kock pouch surgery:

> the change from incontinent to continent is quite dramatic for the human psyche. Being able to have a bath with the continent stoma remains very vivid and satisfying in my mind ... intubating with a large size catheter is sometimes difficult. The bowel tends to become spastic; it has curvatures. If the pouch is full one has to be patient and gently push the well-lubricated catheter in different directions until it reaches the valve and beyond into the pouch ... some foods cause the catheter to plug so extra time is spent in the bathroom flushing it out ... but all things considered the freedom of being bag free outweighs everything. (Kenney 1986)

Few can deny that the quality of life of patients with a satisfactorily functioning Kock pouch is somewhat better than that of patients with a conventional ileostomy (Keighley & Williams 1993). Many patients will, however, need to curtail their lifestyle in order to maintain satisfactory pouch function. Some believe that the morbidity associated with a Kock pouch, that is, pelvic sepsis, pouchitis and nipple valve dysfunction, increases the limitations on lifestyle compared with a Kock pouch and a conventional ileostomy (McLeod & Fazio 1984). It is widely acknowledged that patients who opt for a Kock pouch convey a deep desire to be rid of the incontinent stoma and appliance (Englert & Hass 1986), which in some respects outweighs any associated morbidity. Even when complications occur and the patient may be requested to insert a medina catheter in the pouch long term and hence return to wearing an appliance, this is a psychologically better option in that he or she is aware that this arrangement is potentially not permanent.

McLeod & Fazio (1984) investigated the limitations on normal social activity imposed by a Kock pouch (Table 5.4). Although their study is slightly biased in that the sample used comprised mainly those who had converted from a conventional ileostomy to a Kock pouch, significant results were still highlighted. Limitations in sporting activities, hobbies, work opportunities, clothing and travel were lower in patients with a Kock pouch. Troublesome odour and noise were also less apparent in patients with a continent ileostomy. A Kock pouch should not prevent work or leisure activities. It is envisaged that once the patient has gained confidence with the way in which the pouch functions, normal working capacity and leisure pursuits for that individual can be resumed (Öjerskog et al 1990).

Table 5.4 Quality of life

	Ileostomy ($n = 40$)	Kock pouch ($n = 71$)
Troublesome odour (%)	88	40
Noise (%)	88	34
Thick motion (%)	–	39
Lifestyle limitations		
Diet (%)	54	54
Sports (%)	82	16
Hobbies (%)	49	4
Work (%)	49	13
Clothing (%)	93	13
Travel (%)	49	7

From McLeod & Fazio (1984).

Dietary considerations for the patient with a Kock pouch are dealt with in Chapter 9. In general, however, foods should be enjoyed, eaten in small amounts and chewed well. It should be noted that roughage is more difficult to digest, will require more time when intubating the pouch and will certainly lead to irrigation of the pouch. Daily grape or prune juice will aid in thinning the motion within the pouch, thus improving intubation time and ensuring that irrigation is not necessary on a regular basis.

As with the ileo-anal pouch, a normal sex life for that individual may resume when the patient and partner feel ready. It is well documented that body image changes are less traumatic following a Kock pouch procedure than with a conventional ileostomy (Spencer & Barnett 1982). Male or female sexual dysfunction can occur in anyone who has undergone pelvic surgery. The potential sexual dysfunction that can occur following pouch surgery should be discussed during the preoperative phase. This area is discussed in greater depth in Chapter 10.

It is acknowledged that the contraceptive pill can be recommended as a form of family planning. There is often a fear that it will not be absorbed through the intestinal mucosa and will therefore be ineffective, but this is not the case. If there is an increase in pouch function, an additional contraceptive method will be required.

It is not unreasonable to expect young women of childbearing age to become pregnant following the Kock pouch procedure. As long as there are no underlying gynaecological disorders, becoming pregnant does not appear to be a problem. Throughout the pregnancy, however, the risk of small bowel obstruction and difficulty intubating, as a result of a sliding nipple valve, greatly increases (Curtis et al 1996). Unlike the ileo-anal pouch, vaginal delivery is advocated.

Patients with a Kock pouch are advised to wear or carry some type of medical alert tag or card as the continent ileostomy could easily be mistaken for a conventional stoma. The tag or card should contain the following information:

- Internal pouch/continent ileostomy (Kock pouch)
- Insert medina/ileostomy straight catheter 4–6 hourly (Astra Tech M8371 [sterile] or M8370-5 [non-sterile])
- Do not irrigate

Some patients may also like to make use of the RADAR scheme. After paying a nominal fee, the Kock pouch patient has access to all the disabled toilets in the UK within the scheme. The patient is supplied with a directory of the facilities available for use.

Although the Kock pouch procedure is not advocated as the first surgical option for those with ulcerative colitis or FAP, it does, however, have a place for those patients to whom it is not possible to offer an ileo-anal pouch. Thus, patients still require adequate information in order to make an informed choice, and support must be continued through the rehabilitation period until the patient gains the confidence to maintain a healthy lifestyle, as was enjoyed prior to the initial disease and/or surgery.

CHAPTER 6

The colo-anal pouch and nursing care

ROBIN PHILLIPS AND JULIA WILLIAMS

Colorectal cancer is the most common cancer in non-smoking men and women. When a patient presents with bowel cancer, that cancer is either truly local or else it has already spread elsewhere, usually to the liver. If it has already spread, then, in the absence of very effective systemic chemotherapy, the patient will not be cured. If the tumour is truly local, adequate local surgery will effect a cure, whereas inadequate local surgery will lead to local recurrence.

A patient's survival after colorectal cancer surgery really depends on whether or not microscopic metastases are already present in the liver. These are known as occult hepatic metastases, and, if they are present, the operation will fail to cure the patient. Staging systems, such as Dukes system, simply give an estimate of the chance of occult hepatic metastases already being present: with a Dukes A tumour the chance is low, and 90 per cent of patients are cured; with a Dukes B tumour the chance is moderate, and a cure is achieved in about 60 per cent of cases; and with a Dukes C carcinoma the chance of occult metastases is high, and only about 30–40 per cent are cured (see Chapter 3).

This explains why survival after colorectal cancer surgery is largely outside the surgeon's control: survival depends on whether or not the patient has presented with occult hepatic metastases. This means that there are essentially three desirable surgical end-points: do not kill the patient on the operating table, avoid local recurrence and achieve a good quality of life.

A colonic pouch has a role to play in all three of these areas. Side-to-side anastomoses may be less prone to complications such as anastomotic leak, which leads to death in some patients. The removal of the whole rectum, utilizing total mesorectal excision (TME), is claimed to reduce the local recurrence rate, but it results in a colo-anal anastomosis for most patients with rectal cancer. The construction of a pouch may reduce bowel frequency, thereby enhancing continence and quality of life, and permit the more frequent application of TME.

Total mesorectal excision

The rectum (Figure 6.1) is about 15 cm long and is arbitrarily divided into thirds, each 5 cm long, these being the upper, middle and lower thirds. Cancer of the rectum spreads locally within the wall before spreading to involve adjacent lymph nodes in the rectal mesentery. In most cases, microscopic spread in the rectal wall is less than 2 cm below the palpable lower margin of the tumour, so unless the surgeon is dealing with a poorly differentiated carcinoma, when spread may be as much as 4.5 cm, there is in most cases no surgical reason to remove all of the rectum. By surgeons using modern stapling guns and being aided by better training in deep pelvic dissection, many tumours in the lower third of the rectum can be treated by restorative surgery.

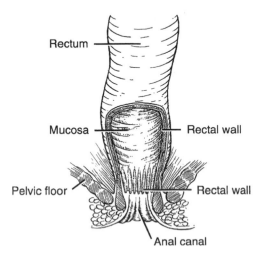

Figure 6.1 Anatomy of the rectum.

In the past, surgeons confronted by cancers in the lower third of the rectum needed to decide whether to perform abdominoperineal excision with a permanent end-colostomy, or proctectomy with colo-anal anastomosis (usually by hand). The problem with such endo-anal colo-anal anastomosis was that function was often initially poor and might take a year or two to improve, if it were going to improve at all (Nicholls et al 1996). The rate of complications, particularly anastomotic leak, was high, so a temporary stoma was usually necessary, and the local recurrence rate started to rise once attempts to restore intestinal continuity low in the pelvis were more frequently applied. Meanwhile, cancers in the middle and upper thirds of the rectum were treated by most surgeons by anterior resection. In the upper third of the rectum, a covering stoma was frequently deemed to be unnecessary.

Over the previous 10 years, however, surgeons have on the whole been persuaded that this approach to rectal cancer surgery results in a higher local recurrence rate than can be achieved by some surgeons who routinely employ TME with colo-anal anastomosis, even for cancers in the middle and sometimes upper third of the rectum.

The rationale for this more extensive surgery lies in the following claims:

- Involved lymph nodes can sometimes be found a few centimetres below the lower palpable margin of the tumour and risk being left behind with conventional surgery.
- The so-called mesorectal envelope is a fragile membrane around the lymph nodes of the rectum, which, if breached, may leak cancer cells from the cut lymphatics into the operative wound, leading to local recurrence, but if kept intact by TME may result in less local recurrence.
- The results of TME are superior to conventional surgical results.

On the other side of the argument, the underlying science is at best dubious, other factors might account for the good surgical results, and colo-anal anastomosis has many complications, almost always needs a defunctioning stoma and has poor function, particularly initially.

The colonic pouch

Initial attempts to create a colonic pouch resulted in a better evacuation frequency but were met with problems of evacuation in a few patients. These seem to have resolved now that much smaller colonic pouches, around 5 cm in length, are being constructed.

A small colonic pouch results in quite good function, bowel actions occurring about twice a day compared with around 4–6 times a day with a straight anastomosis. Nocturnal evacuation is still necessary in about one-third of patients at 2 months, falling to just 11 per cent at 1 year. This is substantially better than the two-thirds nocturnal evacuation at 2 months and 24 per cent at 1 year after colo-anal anastomosis.

The Achilles' heel of the technique remains the problem of evacuation. In one recent study (Hallbrook et al 1996), 10 per cent of patients at 1 year needed regularly to use either suppositories or enemas to achieve evacuation, a proportion that could get worse with time as pouches gradually distend and become floppy.

It therefore seems sensible to consider a colonic pouch in all elderly patients having TME with an anastomosis as they will not be expected to live long enough, either because of their disease or simply because of their age, to be at much risk of pouch decompensation. The situation in young patients is, however, much more difficult. Re-do pelvic surgery, should it prove necessary because of subsequent evacuation difficulties, is problematic and puts the pelvic nerves (Figure 6.2) at risk. Function after a straight colo-anastomosis does improve with time, so there is still an argument that younger patients might do best in the long term without a pouch.

Should the side-to-side anastomosis necessary for colo-pouch anal anastomosis prove to be less likely to leak, this might sway the argument in favour of using colonic pouches in everyone. Whereas one study did claim this, only 2 per cent demonstrating a clinical anastomotic leak with a pouch, compared with 15 per cent with a conventional anastomosis (p <0.03), the groups were very poorly matched for other risk factors for anastomotic leak. Thus, 27 per cent undergoing a straight anastomosis had received preoperative radiotherapy, which might harm healing, compared with only 16% of those receiving a pouch. Similarly, 17 per cent with a pouch were defunctioned and therefore less likely clinically to demonstrate an

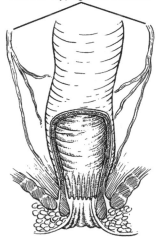

Inferior Hypogastric Nerves

Figure 6.2 Nerves to the rectum.

anastomotic leak, in comparison to 5 per cent acquiring a straight anastomosis.

Patient selection

All cases of carcinoma of the rectum situated in the middle and lower thirds of the rectum and suitable for restorative operation should be considered for TME. There remains, however, some debate over the relative merits of TME in cases of rectal cancer in the upper third of the rectum. Patients with extensive rectal villous adenoma not suited to transanal excision should also be considered for this procedure.

Colo-anal pouch surgery has been described in the treatment of megacolon and megarectum but with little success in view of the slow transit of the gut, which tends to lead to recurrent constipation (Stewart et al 1994).

A colonic pouch might be expected to be performed restoratively in all elderly patients and in all patients whose life expectancy is short. Controversy surrounds the situation with younger patients, despite much of the literature suggesting a significant advantage of the colonic pouch–anal anastomosis over a conventional colo-anal anastomosis in decreasing postoperative bowel frequency and urgency of the neo-rectum (Berger et al 1992, Seow-Choen 1993).

Preoperative considerations

When stoma formation, whether it be temporary or permanent, is contemplated, an anticipation of pain and a threat to lifestyle and body image is likely to occur (Cohen & Lazarus 1982). In order that the patient can begin to come to terms with the surgery and formation of a stoma, preoperative preparation and counselling are necessary.

The patient should ideally be seen by the clinical nurse specialist in stoma care in the outpatient department. This will provide an opportunity for the patient to express fears and concerns with regard to the surgical outcome and lifestyle implications. An explanation of the surgical procedure (including stoma formation) should be provided in verbal, written and diagrammatic ways. As a result of this, the patient will begin to demonstrate understanding, thus working towards adaptation through the process of rehabilitation. It might also be appropriate to involve the Macmillan cancer support nurse at this point.

The preparation of the bowel prior to colonic pouch surgery is similar to that used for any abdominal procedure. At St Mark's Hospital, this constitutes a low-residue diet reducing to free fluids, then clear fluids (whilst taking Picolax) and then nil by mouth 4–6 hours prior to surgery. The use of anticoagulant therapy and anti-embolic stockings is now standard practice.

All patients are seen for the siting of a temporary loop ileostomy, and at this point the clinical nurse specialist in stoma care can reiterate the information relating to the surgical procedure, including the temporary stoma, thus ensuring that the patient has made an informed decision to proceed.

The stoma should be sited carefully, even though it is a temporary one. There is a tendency for loop temporary stomas to be slightly bulky and oval in shape, hence the need to site them with caution. It is widely acknowledged that patients with temporary stomas adapt differently from those with permanent stomas (Wade 1989). It is felt that although the patient has been informed of the rationale underlying the presence of the stoma, that is, to aid the healing process, they usually remain anxious with respect to when the stoma might be closed. Many curtail their lifestyle, insisting that they will resume 'normal' recreational activities once the stoma has been closed. As Wade (1989) highlights, 'the hope of a return to normality, combined with apprehension and dread of going through another operation' provide considerable conflict, which can detract from the patient's rehabilitation.

The preoperative period also allows patients to familiarize themselves with stoma appliances and begin to learn the practicalities of stoma care, thus being introduced to the experiences of living with a temporary loop ileostomy.

The surgical procedure

The patient is catheterized and placed in the Lloyd-Davies position (Figure 6.3), with due care to avoid damage to the lateral popliteal nerve, with resultant foot drop, or undue calf ischaemia from too steep a Trendelenburg position for too long, which can lead to a compartment syndrome, with possible muscular contracture. Some surgeons prefer to use a nasogastric tube, whereas others choose not to.

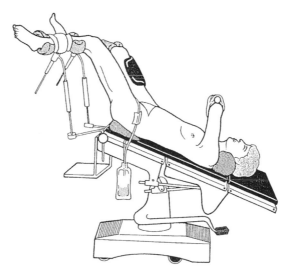

Figure 6.3 The Lloyd-Davies position.

Rectal excision using TME should be performed (Figure 6.4). Experience with ileo-anal pouches in inflammatory bowel disease has taught colorectal surgeons that pouches should never be anastomosed too high up, so pouch–rectal anastomosis should not be carried out.

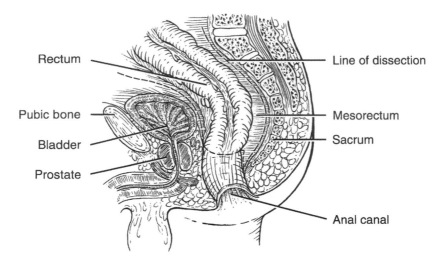

Rectum

Line of dissection

Pubic bone

Mesorectum

Bladder

Sacrum

Prostate

Anal canal

Figure 6.4 Area removed in total mesorectal excision.

Conventionally, surgeons have been advised to use descending colon rather than sigmoid colon for anastomosis because:

- descending colon has a better blood supply than sigmoid colon;
- sigmoid colon generates higher-pressure profiles than descending colon and may contribute to poorer function.

However, an international randomized trial of straight versus pouch anastomosis incidentally used sigmoid colon in 42 per cent of anastomoses without obvious disadvantage. Using sigmoid colon might allow the splenic flexure to be left alone, which could be an advantage in some patients with a high splenic flexure at surgery, but in other circumstances it seems reasonable still to aim to use descending colon for the anastomosis.

A 5 cm pouch (Figure 6.5) can be constructed using one firing of a linear cutter, the pouch then being joined to the anus either by hand transanally or by using a stapling gun, which is much easier. At St Mark's Hospital, a loop ileostomy is used in most cases.

Postoperative care

This should really be no different from care after any major colorectal operation with a covering stoma. Early mobilization should be

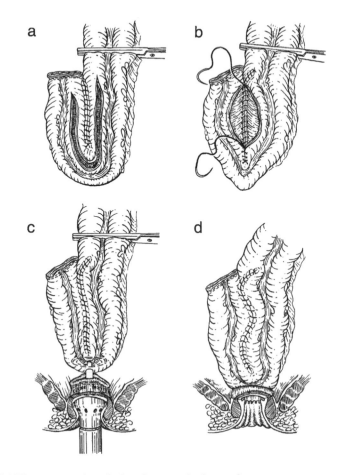

Figure 6.5 The construction of a hand-sewn colonic pouch.

encouraged and fluids and foods introduced when the patient can tolerate them. Stoma care should be taught, and patients can be discharged when able competently to care for themselves, which may be anything from 8 to 12 days postoperatively.

As the patient recovers from surgery, time should be spent teaching self-care of the stoma, with information on how to obtain supplies and dispose of equipment. The physical care of the stoma should be kept as simple as possible. The stoma should be treated like any other area of the body and cleaned with water before being thoroughly dried. A careful examination of the peristomal skin when changing the appliance allows steps to be taken to alleviate any skin problems.

The patient should not leave hospital until he or she is confident about changing the appliance or has some other satisfactory arrangements in place. Dietary advice should include caution concerning foods that may swell in the gut and cause a 'bolus' obstruction, such as sweetcorn and nuts, and foods that may cause more fluid discharge, including salads, vegetables and fruit. An outpatient review at about 6 weeks allows the anastomosis to be felt. It is common for there to be some stenosis, but this can be safely ignored.

Admission for stoma closure should usually be deferred until at least 3 months after the original operation as this allows the immediate postoperative adhesions to be cleared through normal healing processes, which will mean a much easier operation for the surgeon and hopefully fewer complications for the patient. Before stoma closure, a water-soluble contrast X-ray should be taken to rule out any obvious leak from either the pouch itself or the pouch–anal anastomosis. In addition, the pouch and pouch–anal anastomosis should be examined when the patient is anaesthetized, again to check that both sites are satisfactory and to dilate any stenosis.

Long-term expectations

Several studies have reviewed the medium-term functional results of the colonic pouch (Berger et al 1992, Fuchs et al 1998). It has been noted that continence is satisfactory in 96 per cent of patients. The average number of bowel movements in 24 hours is 2–4. Fragmentation of defaecation and urgency are not usually common, but 25 per cent of patients have to use a suppository or an enema to aid evacuation.

Whereas the colonic pouch corrects the loss of reservoir capacity, the transanal colo-anal anastomosis may damage the internal anal sphincter when the anal canal is stretched to complete the anastomosis (Keighley & Williams 1993).

Any surgical intervention carries a certain of risk of complications. Most patients who undergo reconstructive surgery do so to minimize alterations in body ideal, reality and presentation (Price 1990).

The small colonic pouch has been a useful advance when treating rectal cancer patients. It allows the extension of TME to more cases without the concomitant downside of poor function from a low anastomosis, and it should serve to reduce the local recurrence rate. Surgeons may in future find that the side-to-side anastomosis is safe enough to rule out the routine use of a defunctioning stoma, but evidence to date is not sufficiently good for this to be a current recommendation. Concern still surrounds whether pouches will expand and become floppy over time, and because of this worry there should be some hesitation in applying pouches to younger patients, particularly those with benign or early disease.

CHAPTER 7

Continent urinary diversions and rectal bladders

RACHEL LEAVER

History of continent urinary bladders

The oldest form of continent urinary diversion known is the ureterosigmoidostomy (Fisch et al 1992). The idea of diverting urine into the rectum was first described in 1852 by Simon, since when there have been several attempts at updating and improving the technique and overcoming complications to ensure a better outcome for the patient (Wammeck et al 1995). The Mauclaire (1895), the Gersuny (1898), the Heitz-Boyer and the Hovelaque (1912) are all examples of rectal bladders (Wammeck et al 1995). In these pouches, the colon was interrupted and the ureters were implanted into the remaining sigmoid-rectal segment, thus forming a rectal bladder. The patient was given an abdominal (as in the Mauclaire; Figure 7.1) or perineal (for example, the Gersuny, the Heitz-Boyer and the Hovelaque) colostomy. Urine and faeces were therefore kept separate. Continence was achieved by means of the rectal sphincter.

These procedures were unfortunately associated with many complications, most notable of which were nocturnal incontinence, ureteric obstruction, pyelonephritis, renal function deterioration and a high mortality rate. Many of the renal problems were the result of poor technique when re-implanting the ureters. As improvements were made in this area, these problems were eventually resolved, and for the first half of the twentieth century, the modified trans-sigmoid ureterosigmoidostomy was the prime method of urinary diversion (Woodhouse & Christofides 1998) (Figure 7.2).

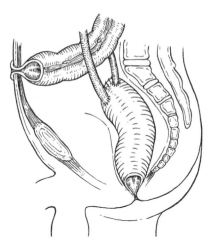

Figure 7.1 The Mauclaire rectal bladder.

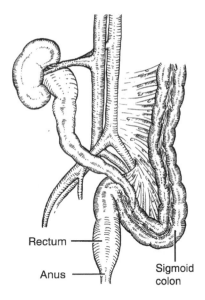

Rectum

Anus

Sigmoid colon

Figure 7.2 An obstructed ureterosigmoidostomy.

Unlike the situation with rectal bladders, urine and faeces are mixed in the ureterosigmoidostomy, and a colostomy is no longer needed as the ureters are directly implanted into the sigmoid colon, the urine and faeces both being evacuated via the anus. The procedure, however, fell out of favour because of persistent complications of infection, electrolyte imbalance, loss of renal function, renal calculi (Fisch et al 1992), the high rate of incontinence especially at night and its poor reputation for morbidity and mortality (Woodhouse & Christofides 1998).

Another concern was the discovery of the incidence of carcinoma at the ureterosigmoid junction in these diversions (Hammer 1929). Initial research showed that the high level of nitrosamine compounds found in the colon (up to 10 times higher than that seen in a normal bladder) might be the causative factor and that it is the presence of both urine and faeces in the bowel that causes the level to rise (Woodhouse 1994). The development of Bricker's ileal conduit in the 1950s, and eventually continent urinary diversions such as the Mitrofanoff or Kock pouch, meant that ureterosigmoidostomy was no longer regarded as the operation of choice.

The development of bladder reconstruction and continent urinary diversion would not have been possible without the research presented by Lapides et al (1972) with regard to intermittent clean self-catheterization. Their findings revolutionized the way in which surgeons approached the diseased bladder and urinary diversion. It allowed them to develop diversions that were more cosmetically pleasing to patients and that also reduced the risk of renal failure and other complications associated with rectal bladders, thus paving the way for the many different types of continent diversion available today.

Continent urinary diversions

There are several different types of continent urinary diversion, for example the Mitrofanoff, the Kock and the Mainz pouches, which rely on different surgical techniques (Kock 1992). The outcome for the patient, regardless of the type of diversion opted for, is the formation of an internal reservoir to contain the urine and a tunnel from this reservoir leading to a continent abdominal stoma. The patient does not have to wear an appliance over this opening, voiding being achieved by inserting a catheter into the stoma and through the tunnel to reach the reservoir (Figure 7.3). Once the pouch is empty, the catheter is removed (Leaver 1994).

Patients requiring a urinary diversion include those with congenital problems, for example bladder exstrophy, or neurological disorders

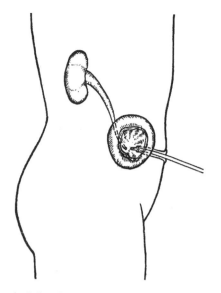

Figure 7.3 Emptying the Mitrofanoff pouch.

such as myelomelingocele that affect the bladder. Other conditions include severe incontinence, cancer and trauma to the bladder. Some patients will have this diversion simply because they find the ileal conduit, ureterosigmoidostomy or rectal bladder unacceptable. Patients should ideally be allowed to decide for themselves which diversion is the optimum solution, although there may be definite reasons why one type of diversion rather than another is deemed more suitable. Factors that should be taken into consideration are:

- medical conditions that will preclude the patient having a lengthy anaesthetic (as surgery may last for 5 hours or more);
- impaired dexterity on the part of the patient;
- a lack of understanding of and commitment to taking care of the diversion postoperatively.

Preoperative patient assessment is vital and should begin during the early stage of the consultation. Patients should be assessed for their mental and physical state as well as their ability to cope with the aftercare. It is important to stress that the care and commitment are for life and that any abuse of the system could lead to serious and sometimes fatal consequences (for example, pouch rupture). It is also

important to assess patients' ability to cope with the very real possibility of complications, which may require more treatment or
surgery.

There is much information for patients to assimilate, and they may
require several sessions to ensure that they fully understand the process
and make the necessary preparations. Compliance and motivation are
therefore as important as physical ability. The patients' carer or partner is ideally included in this assessment, and discharge care-planning
should also start at this point. These operations are rarely performed
as emergencies, so patients have time to plan for family and work
commitments as well as to undergo a thorough preoperative assessment by the nurse specialist allocated to look after them. The recovery
period from this surgery may be quite lengthy (the minimum being
about 3 months), especially if there are complications. Patients should
therefore also be encouraged to make arrangements for their aftercare
once they have been discharged home.

Patients are usually in hospital for 2–3 weeks. A period of up to 4
weeks at home follows as the catheterizing tunnel can take 6 weeks to
heal before it is safe enough to remove the catheter without any
danger of the tunnel rapidly closing over. The patient is then re-
admitted to have the catheters removed and to learn to catheterize
and care for the pouch.

Preoperative care

The findings of preoperative investigations such as kidney function,
bladder pressure and blood tests allow the surgeon to determine
what type of reconstruction is suitable for the patient and to form a
baseline set of readings against which to compare any postoperative
and follow-up test results (Leaver 1997).

Stoma siting

On admission for surgery, it is important, besides undertaking the
usual preoperative care (for example, clearing the bowel), to site the
stoma correctly. The prime concern is to position it where it will be
discrete (such as in the right iliac fossa or the umbilicus). The patient
must also be able to see and reach the stoma and be able to catheterize it easily. Even though no appliance needs to be used over the
stoma, it is still advisable to try to choose a site that avoids folds and

creases in the skin. As with conventional stomas, it is also wise to mark the stoma site when the patient is clothed (Fillingham 1997) and in the position in which he or she will undertake catheterization, for example sitting in a wheelchair (Leaver 1997).

Postoperative care

Patients may require a short stay in intensive care immediately post-operatively. Besides the usual care, the most important aspect is the care of the catheters and tubes draining urine from the new pouch or bladder (Figure 7.4). The pouch itself must not be allowed to stretch before it has properly healed. Care must also be taken that the Mitrofanoff catheter is safely anchored in place. These catheters must be flushed with 20 ml of sterile saline twice daily to keep them free of mucus and debris. After the first 4 postoperative days, the new pouch has healed sufficiently that it can be regularly washed out (using two 50 ml batches of saline twice a day).

Once the patient can tolerate fluids, he or she should be encouraged to drink at least 2–3 litres a day. Drinking cranberry juice twice daily, or taking the equivalent in capsule form (available from health food shops), also helps to reduce the risk of urinary infection (Avorn et al 1994) and the amount of mucus produced (Rosenbaum et al 1989, Leaver 1996a).

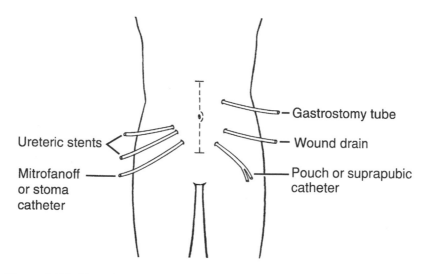

Figure 7.4 Position of catheters and drainage tubes.

Discharge

Patients are discharged home with the Mitrofanoff catheter and often the suprapubic catheter in situ. The time spent at home not only allows them to recover from the surgery, but also helps them to gain confidence in handling catheters and urine drainage bags; it gives patients back some control over their body and helps them to become accustomed to the workings of their new bladder. This is good preparation for the final tubes being removed and catheterization starting.

Patients should be instructed to:

- ensure that their catheters are draining at all times;
- wash out the pouch at least twice daily;
- ensure that, should the tunnel catheter inadvertently fall out, it is replaced as soon as possible to prevent the stoma permanently closing.

They should also be warned that a urinary infection or/and catheter site infection is almost inevitable and that, should one occur, a urine specimen and/or swabs should be taken by the general practitioner, who may prescribe a course of antibiotics. Most patients will need the services of a district nurse to help with dressings and ensure both that the catheters are in place and draining, and that the patient is coping. Referral to a local stoma nurse or continence advisor for support is also advisable. Patients and their carers must be reassured that they can contact the hospital at any time if they are at all worried.

Re-admission

Patients are usually re-admitted for 2–3 nights, although this varies and should really be dictated by the patient. Discharge home should only be considered when the patient is happy and confident with his or her ability to catheterize the pouch.

Expanding the pouch

The pouch should not be expanded too quickly as this can be painful and may cause damage if it is allowed to become too full too soon. A 2–3 hourly catheterization regime when there is a volume of urine of 150–250 ml is usually well tolerated by most patients, although this may of course vary, and some patients may have to empty more frequently. Patients should be reassured that, as the pouch expands, they will be able to catheterize less frequently. Most patients eventually catheterize their pouch between four to six times a day depending on the volume it holds, what sensations they have and how much they drink. It is vital that the pouch is not allowed to overfill. This may lead to the patient being unable to push the catheter into the tunnel to empty the pouch and/or the pouch rupturing.

Emptying the pouch at night

It is advisable to instruct patients to set an alarm clock to wake them up at least once a night for the first few weeks to empty their pouch. Many patients eventually manage to sleep the whole night through because the pouch expands to hold a much larger volume (400–500 ml or more) of urine. Restricting fluid intake before bed-time also helps by reducing the amount of urine produced at night. Some patients may of course have enough sensation in their pouch to wake up spontaneously.

Catheterization

The catheters used are usually male-length PVC Nelaton type intermittent catheters, which are free on prescription (because the Mitrofanoff opening is still classed as a stoma). Catheterization of the stoma follows the same principles as clean intermittent urethral self-catheterization (Table 7.1).

The size of catheter used varies, but it is usually either a size 12 ch or 14 ch. There are a variety of catheters available, both pre-lubricated and non-lubricated, and patients may need to try various types until they find the one which best suits their needs. It is advisable to use a water-based lubricating jelly such as KY with the non-lubricated catheters. Many patients prefer to dispense with using this after a while.

Catheter care

Many non-pre-lubricated catheters are re-usable, but it is advisable to check the recommendations of the individual manufacturers.

Table 7.1: Continent urinary pouches: patient guidelines

How do I catheterize my pouch?
- Please remember that this is a clean procedure. Make sure you have everything you need with you before you start to wash your hands. This avoids the unnecessary handling of equipment and potential contamination, which could introduce infection into the pouch
- Assume a comfortable position by either sitting on the toilet, standing over the toilet or sitting on a chair or in your wheelchair
- If you wish, lubricate your catheter with lubricating jelly to ease its insertion
- Insert the catheter gently until urine begins to flow
- When the flow has stopped, try pushing the catheter in a little further – you may find that more urine will flow out
- When you think your pouch is empty, rotate the catheter gently as you withdraw it. This may dislodge any debris or mucus blocking the tube and allows more urine to flow
- If you experience pain on inserting the catheter, do not push it in any further

Patients re-using their catheters are advised to wash them out in hot soapy water after use, dry them carefully and store them in a watertight container such as a plastic freezer bag. Catheters should never be left soaking in a sterilizing or disinfecting solution as this encourages bacterial growth.

It is a good idea to encourage patients to ensure that they have spare catheters and washing-out equipment at work, at school, in the car, at friends' or relatives' houses and so on as well as at home in case they forget or mislay their catheter. This will ensure that they will always be able to empty their pouch.

Care of the stoma

Most patients do not cover their stoma site, especially if it is in the umbilicus, but it is wise to warn patients that they may experience slight leakage via the stoma at first while the pouch expands and the new system settles down. Some patients will always ooze mucus via the stoma and may prefer to cover it with gauze to save soiling their clothes. It is advisable to use a waterproof dressing over the site when swimming to protect the stoma from contamination from the sea or swimming pool water, although it is perfectly safe to bath or shower without any covering.

The aim is to discharge the patients home when:

- they are confident that they are able to identify when they need to empty the pouch;
- they are able to catheterize the pouch competently and empty it completely;
- they have absorbed all the information they need to cope with any problems that they may encounter.

This knowledge should be backed up with written information for both the patient and any carers to use as a reference.

Aftercare

Because of the complexity of the surgery and the potential for problems to arise, the rate of complications can be as high as 20 per cent (Woodhouse & Gordon 1994), so it is important to follow these patients up rigorously. Follow-up should include X-rays and ultrasound examinations of the kidneys and pouches, kidney function tests, blood tests, blood pressure measurements, urine tests and bladder pressure tests. These might detect the causes of the more common complications (Woodhouse 1994) such as:

- incontinence
- stenosis of the stoma
- urinary infection
- metabolic acidosis
- stone formation
- renal damage.

It is essential to ensure that the system remains a low-pressure one, in order to protect the upper urinary tract, whilst being compliant enough to hold a reasonable volume of urine, staying continent and being easy to catheterize. Patients may have to undergo further surgery to achieve this. They should be advised to wear a medical bracelet or pendant in case of emergency.

The successful outcome of surgery relies on the combined efforts of the hospital-based surgeons and nurses and community carers, as well as care, commitment and compliance on the part of the patients

themselves. Despite the high maintenance and the very real possibility of complications and repeated surgery, most patients are happy to
comply and feel it is a small price to pay to have an internal system of
which they are in control, which does not need an appliance and
which helps them in their quest to feel 'normal' (Leaver 1998).

Rectal bladders: the Mainz sigmoid II pouch

Unfortunately, all urinary diversions have a high complication rate.
Woodhouse & Chistofides (1998) state that, in practice, it seems that
the more complicated the system, the higher the rate of complications. The psychological impact of these diversions is also a problem
for some patients. The difficulty people have in accepting a conventional stoma has been well documented, but it is important to be
aware that there are some patients who find the intermittent self-
catheterization of a continent stoma such as the Mitrofanoff
completely unacceptable or physically impossible. These patients
may not comply with the care that such diversions need, which could
lead to severe problems. A different approach is clearly needed for
such patients, and rectal bladders may once again offer a more
acceptable alternative.

Many of the renal complications associated with rectal bladders
have been solved by improvements in ureteric re-implantation, and
hyperchloraemic metabolic acidosis and electrolyte imbalance can
now be controlled. These developments, plus improvements in techniques of bowel preparation, antibiotic therapy and absorbable suture
materials, have led surgeons to look again at modified ureterosigmoidostomy as an alternative (appliance-free) continent diversion.

Surgeons have also applied the knowledge gained when dealing
with enterocystoplasties and continent pouches over the past few
decades to the problems encountered in the past with ureteric reflux
and pyelonephritis (Woodhouse & Christofides 1998). These problems were found to be the result of high-pressure peristalsis in the
bowel. Coffey (1911) showed that it was the high rectal pressure that
caused the reflux of faeces into the kidneys. To overcome this pressure, the bowel must be detubularized. The rectum is opened longi-
tudinally and closed transversely to form a pouch, the ureters being
implanted into this pouch, which remains continuous with
the sigmoid colon (Figures 7.5 and 7.6). This pouch is called the

sigma-rectum pouch or Mainz sigmoid II pouch and was described by Fisch and Hohenfellner in 1991. The procedure results in two main changes:

- the elimination of mass contractions and high pressure peaks in the colon;
- an increase in the volume that the reservoir can hold.

This modified rectal pouch acts as a reservoir, allowing the patient to hold urine until ready to void. In time, patients learn how to differentiate between needing to pass urine and having their bowels open even though both events happen via the rectum.

Preoperative care

The input by the stoma nurse or continence adviser at this stage is invaluable to assess the patient during preparation for surgery. Patients tend to focus on the fact that an appliance will not be needed and that voiding will be more 'normal' than with a conduit or continent pouch. This may blind the patient to the potential complications of the surgery and the impact on their subsequent lifestyle.

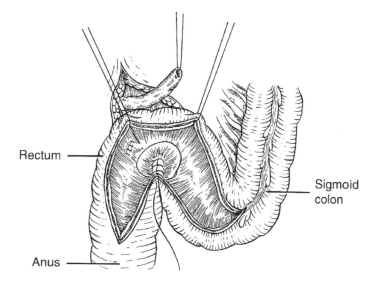

Figure 7.5 Opening of anterior wall of the bowel.

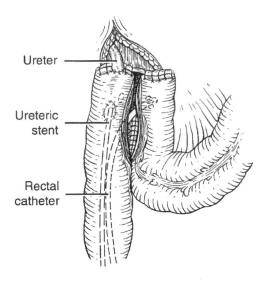

Figure 7.6 Closure of the anterior pouch wall.

Patients should be warned that the mixture of urine and faeces might produce a strong smell, which may be offensive and therefore unacceptable to both them and members of their household. Considerations related to, for example, separate bathrooms and the problems associated with emptying the pouch in public facilities should also be discussed (Leaver 1997).

All rectal bladders require patients to have a competent anal sphincter in order to avoid becoming doubly incontinent postoperatively. The competence of the anal sphincter is therefore of paramount importance. Fisch (1992) recommends that patients need to be able to hold a 300 ml water enema for 3–4 hours without leaking. This test, together with rectodynamic evaluations, which should include an anal sphincter profile, will establish whether continence will be possible after the operation. Alternatively, a sloppy 'porridge' enema may be used instead of the water enema to imitate more closely the contents of the rectum postoperatively (Leaver 1997).

Postoperative care

Patients are usually in hospital for 2 or 3 weeks and require the same preoperative preparation as for any procedure of reconstructive surgery involving the use of bowel. Postoperatively, the rectal bladder is kept empty of urine and faeces to allow the anastomosis to heal. One or two ureteric stents and a rectal catheter are left in situ to drain the rectal pouch. Many patients find this part of the procedure uncomfortable because all the tubes emerge via the anus to be attached to drainage bags. This makes it very difficult to find a comfortable position when lying or sitting.

The rectal catheter is flushed twice daily with sterile saline (20–30 ml) to keep it patent. This is important as urine will initially drain via the ureteric stents, and the catheter can therefore become blocked with solid matter. The patient may also have one or two wound drains. These, however, usually emerge via the abdomen.

Voiding

The stents are removed approximately 10 days post-surgery, the rectal catheter being removed 24–48 hours later. Patients need a lot of support, encouragement and reassurance at this stage. Many experience frequency and incontinence, and they should be encouraged to wear pads for the first few weeks until they have gained more control. Patients should be taught how to expand their rectal bladder by attempting to resist the urge to empty it for an increasingly longer period of time. As the bladder stretches, the volume of urine it can hold will increase, and continence will also improve. The skin around the anus should be protected with a barrier cream to minimize irritation by urine and faeces should the anal sphincter leak.

Most patients eventually void every 2–4 hours by day, and some may have to wake to empty at night. This depends on the size of the pouch, what sensation they have and how much they drink, varying from patient to patient. In the author's experience, it may take patients up to 3 months to establish a regular voiding pattern and to overcome problems with incontinence.

Common complications

Incontinence (predominantly nocturnal) may continue for the first weeks and even months post-surgery. Patients report that they can pass wind but only after they have emptied the pouch of urine.

Hyperchloraemic acidosis is still a potential problem, although Woodhouse & Christofides (1998) have found that this does not seem to be a problem in the early postoperative period. They attribute this to the fact that urine does not drain in a retrograde manner into the rest of the colon, so the surface area available for the transfer of ions is less than that seen in other diversions.

Of course, the threat remains of secondary malignancy following the Mainz II procedure because of the high risk posed by the mixture of faeces and urine in the bowel. Neoplasia usually manifests itself 20–30 years post-surgery (Stewart 1986), and patients will need meticulous yearly endoscopic follow-up from the twelfth postoperative year to ensure the early detection of any tumour forming in the pouch (Fisch et al 1992, Woodhouse & Christofides 1998).

The Mainz sigma II procedure is relatively simple to perform, and many of the problems encountered in the past, such as ureteric reflex, have been resolved. It has the added advantage of allowing the patient to void spontaneously without the need for an appliance. This makes the Mainz II pouch an attractive alternative for patients and heralds the resurgence of the rectal bladder as another option for patients needing a urinary diversion.

CHAPTER 8

Controversies and problem-solving with regard to ileo-anal pouches

JULIA WILLIAMS AND R. JOHN NICHOLLS

Restorative proctocolectomy aims to improve quality of life by avoiding a permanent ileostomy and thus allowing patients to defaecate in the normal way. Some studies have reported a satisfactory quality of life after restorative proctocolectomy (Sagar et al 1993), whereas others have challenged the notion of such improvements (Kohler & Troidl 1995). Whatever one's personal view of patients' quality of life following restorative procedures, it is evident that ileo-anal pouch surgery is being performed more and more in patients with ulcerative colitis and familial adenomatous polyposis (FAP) (Figure 8.1).

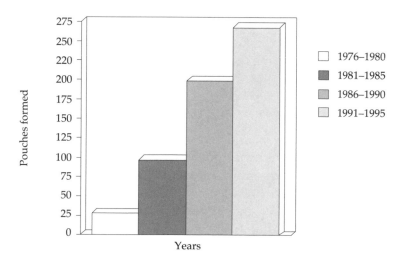

Figure 8.1 Number of cases of ileo-anal pouch surgery at St Mark's for ulcerative colitis and familial adenomatous polyposis.

143

From the literature, it is evident that the hallmark of a good pouch is based upon its function and whether the patient remains continent of faeces and/or free of leakage of mucus (Lewis et al 1993), but anecdotal evidence suggests that although patients may have good pouch function, lifestyle constraints to achieve this may be considerable. Almost every step of the operation has become the subject of some degree of controversy. This has arisen partly to make the operation technically easier and partly to achieve the best function with a minimum of complications.

However hard the surgeon tries, the procedure has a fairly high complication rate. Mortality, however, is very low indeed, and despite complications and an uncertain long-term future for the operation, it is now the most frequently employed procedure in the surgical treatment of ulcerative colitis (Keighley 1996; Keighley et al 1987). Many of the complications are minor but in some way threaten the success of the procedure. The main complications causing concern include pelvic sepsis, usually associated with a degree of breakdown of the ileo-anal anastomosis, intestinal obstruction and fistulation from the anastomosis or the reservoir itself to the exterior, usually to the abdominal wall. It is clear that the operation can be accomplished by various different technical adaptations of a common theme, some of these differences being controversial.

In this chapter, an attempt will be made to discuss the controversies and problems most pertinent to the patient with an ileo-anal pouch. An understanding of these will enable the nurse caring for the patient to have the knowledge and skills to provide care and practical support during the patient's recovery and/or adaptation to living with a pouch.

Patient selection and satisfaction

The first point to be considered prior to any surgical procedure is case selection. There are no apparent criteria for this within the literature apart from the predisposing condition and good anal sphincter control (Pezim & Nicholls 1985a). It has been suggested that the patient's psychological state and motivation should also be considered (Nemer & Rolstad 1985), but in practice it would seem that these latter points are often ignored.

Hull & Erwin-Toth (1996) suggest that although most patients with ulcerative colitis and FAP are 'excellent candidates for the pelvic pouch procedure, careful pre-operative assessment is needed to ensure good results. Oresland (1996) indicates that when the patient is counselled preoperatively, thought must be given to the fact that whatever decision the patient is likely to make, it will ultimately have a profound impact on the rest of his or her life. It is therefore of the utmost importance that the option chosen is the correct and optimal operation for that particular patient. There appears to be little emphasis on this point within the literature reviewed, but what is suggested is suitability for pouch surgery.

It is evident that patients in whom this procedure is contraindicated are those suffering from Crohn's disease, anal sphincter incompetence or a low rectal carcinoma (Taylor et al 1994). Phillips (1991) warns, however, that the colitic patient 'with an aversion to hospitals, an encyclopaedic knowledge of public conveniences and a simple desire just to be well, may undergo major pouch surgery; only to find urgency, frequency and regular outpatient attendance', thus bringing about little change. Similarly, the patient with FAP, who has had a relatively normal bowel habit, may now find the alteration disturbing (Taylor et al 1994). Other relative contraindications include age, obesity, malnutrition, sepsis, long-term steroid therapy and immunosuppresive therapy (Nemer & Rolstad 1985).

Much of the literature on patient selection refers to physiological contraindications, paying little attention to how the patient might withstand the functional management of the pouch, bearing in mind that the function and adaptation of the pouch can be slow. As pouch function gradually improves, some patients find that they are unable to resume the activities enjoyed prior to their illness and surgery as quickly as they had anticipated (Bond et al 1997).

Nemer & Rolstad (1985) suggest that patients 'with significant emotional or psychological history should be considered only with extreme caution', highlighting also that, since the long-term results of pouch procedures remain unknown, patients in whom non-compliance is predictable should not be offered this procedure as an option. Probert et al (1993) indicate that the consequences of restorative proctocolectomy should be discussed objectively and in depth so that the patient contemplating such surgery can make an informed decision about the choice of surgery. Anecdotally, it would appear that these issues are sometimes forgotten, and it is only with hindsight that thought prevails. Taylor et al (1994), however, stress that 'it cannot be overemphasised that to reap the best results from restorative proctocolectomy, patients' motivation and commitment must be total'.

As previously highlighted, 'restorative proctocolectomy is here to stay' (Keighley 1996). Patients clearly want it, despite the fact that there is quite a high complication rate and an uncertain long-term future for the operation (Bond et al 1997). 'The most vocal advocates of continent procedures are the patients themselves' (Salter 1992a). Oresland (1996) implies that the great attraction of the ileo-anal pouch is that 'these patients use their normal route of defaecation'. Salter (1992a) highlights that the reasons most commonly cited for having an ileo-anal pouch include 'greater confidence, ease of management and the feeling of being normal'. Fujita et al (1992) suggest that satisfaction with the operation is 'closely related to confidence with regard to physical strength and the ability to manage frustration'.

In a recent survey by Bond et al (1997) regarding patients' perspectives of life with an ileo-anal pouch, 72 per cent of respondents who had had an ileostomy were asked whether or not they would have preferred to keep it, the pouch being overwhelmingly seen as preferable. In contrast, Awad et al (1993) highlighted that 87 per cent of patients with a permanent ileostomy, when asked, stated that they would prefer to keep the ileostomy in preference to an ileo-anal pouch.

A recent longitudinal study (Marcello et al 1993) showed that 94 per cent of the 428 respondents were satisfied with their ileo-anal pouch and would recommend the procedure to others contemplating such surgery. Those who were not pleased with the outcome of their pouch suggested that prospective patients should consider all options available to them.

An audit conducted by Keighley et al (1993) highlighted that, over a period of 9 years, about 10 per cent of their pouch procedures failed, resulting in the removal of the pouch. These authors stated that over half of these failures were were caused by patients' dissatisfaction with the functional results of their pouch. Keighley et al (1993) stressed that had preoperative patient selection been somewhat more detailed, pouch formation might in some cases not have been performed, thus ultimately preventing eventual excision. Even though such concepts as eventual satisfaction and expectation are

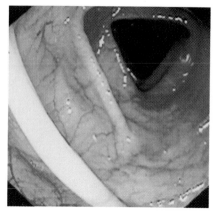

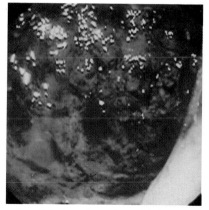

Plate 1 Colonoscopic appearance of normal transverse colon in a patient with left-sided colitis.

Plate 2 Active ulcerative colitis in sigmoid colon (same patient as above).

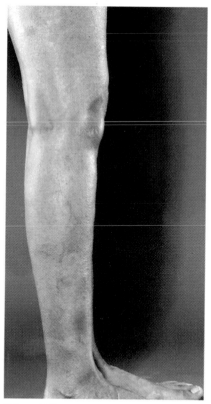

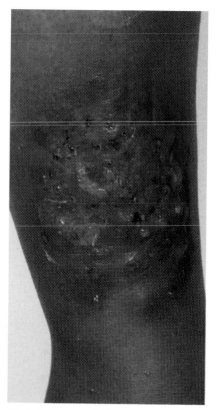

Plate 3 The multiple raised red lesions of erythema nodosum on the legs in patient with active ulcerative colitis.

Plate 4 Characteristic appearances of pyoderma gangrenosum on the leg of a patient with active ulcerative colitis; note the colouration, the pus and the undermining of the ulcer edges; the beginnings of the cribiform scarring are also apparent.

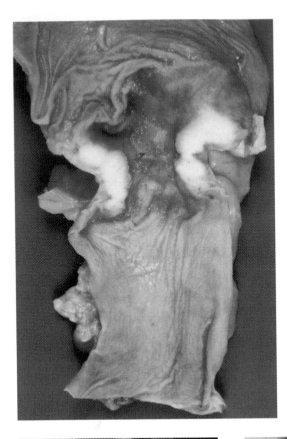

Plate 5 Adenocarcinoma of the rectum.

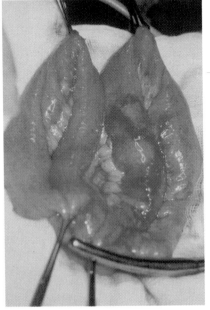

(a)

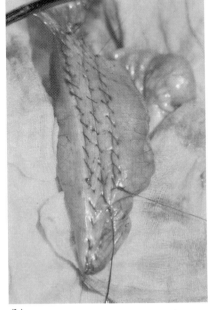

(b)

Plates 6 a, b Ileo-anal pouch construction.

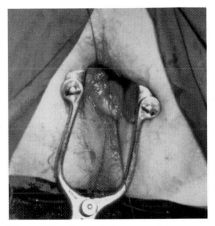

Plate 7 Pouch anal anastomosis.

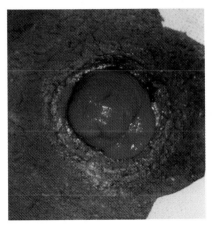

Plate 9 Loop ileostomy.

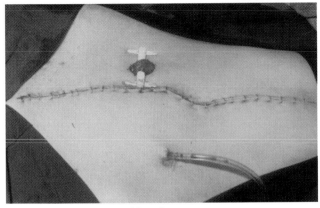

Plate 8 Loop ileostomy with rod.

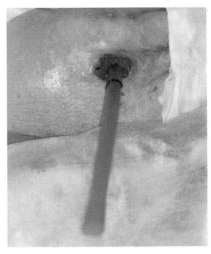

Plate 10 The medina catheter in situ.

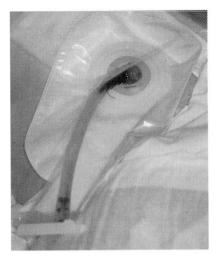

Plate 11 Medina in pouch with stoma appliance.

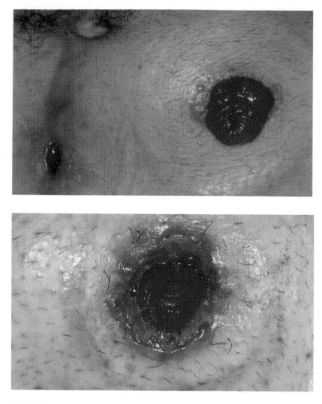

Plate 12
End-ileostomy and
mucous fistula.

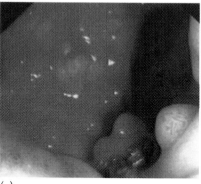

Plate 13 Mucosal
separation with
stomal retraction.

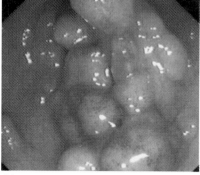

(a)

(b)

Plate 14 a, b, c: Juvenile polyps. Many
polyps can be seen in the upper, mid and
lower rectum, requiring this 14-year-old
girl to undergo a colectomy and pouch
procedure.

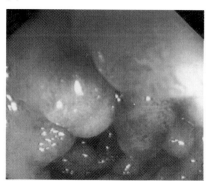

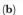

(c)

difficult to quantify and even define, it seems that very little is documented within the surgical literature, the subjective feelings of the patients thus being neglected (Sagar et al 1993).

Fujita et al (1992) identified that those who had suffered with ulcerative colitis were more satisfied with their pouch function and surgical outcome than those with FAP. The authors felt that this difference bore a close relationship to the personality factors of ego and strength. They also highlighted that all patients with either disease who defaecated less than three times a day and had no nocturnal motions and no soiling showed complete satisfaction with their pouch status and operation. In contrast, patients defaecating more than seven times a day or more than once per week nocturnally, and soiling more than four times weekly, demonstrated high frustration and were dissatisfied. Fujita et al (1992) concluded that satisfaction with surgery correlated not only with objective outcome, but also with personality and lifestyle.

Crohn's disease

It is widely acknowledged that restorative procedures are most suited to those with ulcerative colitis or FAP; restorative proctocolectomy has for some time been considered to be quite inappropriate for patients with Crohn's disease. Kock pouches were originally constructed for both Crohn's disease and ulcerative colitis. It is recognized that patients are in some cases selected for pouch surgery with a preoperative diagnosis of ulcerative colitis that later turns out to be indeterminate colitis or Crohn's disease. Studies have shown that if recurrence occurs, it often arises away from the pouch rather than within it (Hyman et al 1991). Although pouches are excised as a result of the presence of Crohn's disease, the complication rates are equal to those of any surgical procedure for Crohn's disease resulting in an anastomosis (Fazio & Church 1988).

Panis et al (1996) have proposed that selected patients with Crohn's disease can be offered a pouch provided the disease is confined to the large bowel with sparing of the anus and small intestine. It might well be questioned whether this diagnosis is in actual fact indeterminate colitis, for which many patients are offered restorative procedures.

It has been suggested that comparing pouch surgery in Crohn's disease with pouch surgery in ulcerative colitis is not appropriate and that the choice of surgery for Crohn's disease should be made on the basis of the distribution of the disease (Phillips 1998). It is rare, however, to encounter cases of Crohn's disease with rectal inflammation without anal disease. Indeed, some of these may be examples of indeterminate colitis in which there are features of both ulcerative colitis and Crohn's disease. On the whole, indeterminate colitis patients have a lower failure rate than those with Crohn's disease. The fact remains, however, that failure in patients with Crohn's disease remains high, at between about 20 and 40% (Hyman et al 1991), and except in exceptional circumstances, it is most unwise to offer the operation to patients with Crohn's disease.

The surgical procedure

Most surgeons consider that the main purpose of creating an internal pouch for patients is to cure disease while improving quality of life. Several controversies exist amongst surgeons over the best possible way to achieve this, much of which lies within the surgical procedure itself.

Proctocolectomy aims to eliminate the risk of colon cancer in patients with FAP or long-standing ulcerative colitis, but some controversy exists over the optimal time for surgery. The dispute rests between the boundaries of the medical and surgical treatments, although obviously if the patient presents with any degree of dysplasia, surgery must unquestionably be instituted. Probert et al (1993) identified that a high colectomy rate is unnecessary and may prejudice survival. Indeed, it suggests that attention should be focused on which patients really need a colectomy rather than which restorative procedure they should undergo.

It has been suggested that, during the phase of colonic dissection, division of the blood vessels should be made proximally in order to achieve a radical regional lymphovascular clearance. This would cover the eventuality of an unrecognized carcinoma, but no information is as yet able to prove that this step is useful. However, provided a patient with ulcerative colitis has had a preoperative colonoscopy carried out by a competent practitioner, it is unlikely, albeit not impossible, that an invasive carcinoma or dysplasia would be missed. It would thus seem common sense to widen the clearance where dysplasia is known to be present. In FAP, this would apply to patients with large adenomas in which there might be a malignant focus.

Although rectal dissection is now the standard procedure in patients with ulcerative colitis, some debate surrounds whether the distal bowel should be bought to the surface of the abdomen as a mucous fistula (Figure 8.2 and Plate 12) or closed and left within the abdomen. A mucous fistula is often difficult for the patient to manage because it is usually sited within the lower aspect of the midline incision, it lies flush with the skin and the exudate varies considerably; above all, however, the patient is not usually prepared for it to be there.

The decision of whether it is safer to close the distal end of the bowel is made at the time of operation: the general condition of the patient and the state of the bowel wall will determine this. It seems reasonable to close the stump if toxicity and malnutrition are minimal and there is no great oedema of the bowel. Otherwise, a mucous fistula should be regarded as the safer method of managing the distal bowel.

When a three-stage procedure is advocated and the patient has previously been treated by colectomy with ileostomy and preservation of a low rectal stump, it can be difficult safely to identify and dissect the rectum. With a low division, the anterior structure tends to fall back posteriorly, and scarring will make access to the rectal stump difficult. In males, there is a danger of damaging the seminal

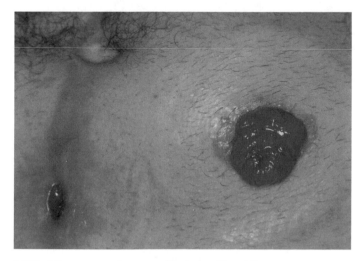

Figure 8.2 End-ileostomy and mucous fistula (see Plate 12).

vesicles and the autonomic nerves in the rectoprostatic septum; in females, the vagina is at risk. The consequence in both cases may be direct damage to these organs, encouraging fistulation to the ileo-anal anastomosis if pelvic sepsis occurs postoperatively.

In patients with known rectal carcinoma or ulcerative colitis with dysplasia, dissection should be carried out in the presacral space with a full removal of the mesorectum. The difficulty here is the incidence of postoperative urinary and sexual dysfunction. Much of the literature suggests this incidence is minimal (Sagar et al 1993) and that if dysfunction does occur, it is temporary.

Type of reservoir

More has been written on the type of reservoir (Figure 8.3) than on any other technical aspect of restorative proctocolectomy. When the ileo-anal pouch procedure was first described, it was asked whether a

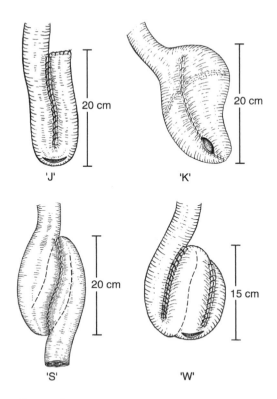

Figure 8.3 Types of reservoir.

reservoir was actually necessary. Ravitch & Sabiston (1947) demonstrated good results in two cases of proctocolectomy and straight ileo-anal anastomosis. Subsequent experience with this procedure showed, however, that a high frequency of defaecation, including night evacuation and urgency, was common. Several studies since then have proved that forming a reservoir provides a level of frequency with continence that is acceptable to the patient (Martin et al 1977).

In the original description of the ileo-anal pouch procedure by Parks & Nicholls (1978), a three-loop or 'S' shaped reservoir was advocated. Over 50 per cent of their initial patients needed to use a catheter to aid the evacuation of the pouch (Nicholls & Lubowski 1987), but with subsequent modifications in pouch design, catheterization has become almost a thing of the past. Most surgeons choose to construct a 'J' (two-looped) (Utsunomiya et al 1980) or 'W' (four-looped) (Nicholls & Lubowski 1987) reservoir in which there is no efferent ileal limb, which was the main factor responsible for the failure of spontaneous evacuation.

The 'J' design is simple to construct using staples and is the most widely used configuration, whereas the 'W' design is more complex even though it has the advantage of greater capacity. Which design is used depends on the surgeon's preference. The suggestion is that the larger the capacity, the better the function of the pouch will be. Some surgeons feel, however, that a spherically shaped 'J' pouch can provide as good a function as a 'W' pouch, simultaneously using less small intestine (Table 8.1).

Table 8.1 Comparison of function for different pouch configurations

	S (58)	J (21)	W (108)	K (26)
Frequency per 24 hours (+/- mean)	3.6 +/- 1.4	5.5 +/- 1.4	4.0 +/- 1.1	4.9 +/- 1.5
Night >1 per night per week (%)	21	57	23	62
Medication (%)	10	57	23	69
Continence				
Normal	44	17	93	15
Minor leak	12	3	13	11
Faecal leak	2	1	2	0

Reporting a comparison of frequency of defaecation between 'S', 'J' and 'W' shaped reservoirs, Pezim & Nicholls (1985a) observed an inverse relationship between the frequency of defaecation and the maximum tolerated volume of the reservoir as measured by the inflation of a balloon introduced into the pouch through the anus. This would thus suggest that capacity is a factor determining frequency. From the literature, it would appear that it does not really matter what configuration of pouch is made as long as it is large enough (Tuckson & Fazio 1991). It is well recognized that, with time, pouch volume increases following the closure of the ileostomy.

Function can be divided into the components of frequency, urgency, continence and need for anti-diarrhoeal medication. An important aspect of frequency is the occurrence of night-time evacuation. Diurnal frequency may well be affected by various factors, including micturition, habit and consciousness of bowel function, but at night these do not apply. Nobody would willingly get up at night unless forced to do so; therefore night evacuation provides a more sensitive guide of function than overall 24 hour frequency. The need for anti-diarrhoeal medication may also be a sensitive guide to function.

Mucosectomy

Another area of controversy is whether or not a mucosectomy should be carried out. The term 'mucosectomy' refers to the removal of the epithelial lining at the top of the anal canal down to the level of the dentate line (Figure 8.4). The mucosa in question refers to the transitional zone and contains sensory receptors.

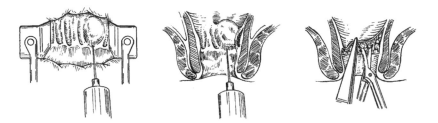

Figure 8.4 Endo-anal mucosectomy.

The reason for undertaking mucosectomy is to ensure the completeness of excision of the disease itself. The concern regards the incidence of dysplasia in the mucosa within the anal canal in patients suffering from both ulcerative colitis and FAP. King et al (1989) reported the findings of 16 consecutive patients with ulcerative colitis. Of these, four had moderate dysplasia of the anal mucosa, and in one case there was a poorly differentiated carcinoma. This demonstrates that the anal canal is not entirely free of the risk of malignant change. In the case of FAP, it is obligatory to undertake a mucosectomy because of the nature of predisposing malignant disease.

In addition to this, if mucosectomy is undertaken with a double-stapled pouch–anal anastomosis, there is an increased risk of cuffitis, there being evidence that this can cause significant pouch dysfunction in some patients (Thompson-Fawcett et al 1999). Studies show that when there is evidence of inflammation within the pouch, it is more severe in its distal than its proximal zones (Setti Carraro et al 1998).

Stapled versus hand-sewn anastomosis

Many surgeons prefer to staple the pouch–anal anastomosis as this speeds up the procedure, whereas others continue to hand-sew. The stapling of a 'W' shaped pouch during its construction can, as a result of the difference between the ileo-anal anastomosis and the pouch, prove to be a difficult procedure, so hand-sewing is preferable.

Those surgeons who do use a stapling technique do so in order to preserve the anal transitional zone and prevent the stretching of the anal sphincter. The main aim is to achieve an anastomosis at the level of the anorectal junction. There is some evidence to suggest that if a double 'J' shaped pouch is stapled, it may be difficult to achieve a precise anastomosis at the anorectal junction, hence leaving a slightly longer stump than is desired as a result of the stapling (Slors et al 1995). Consequently, for the patient, this may result in a retained rectal stump, leading to evacuation difficulties as well as some residual inflamed mucosa.

A further disadvantage of stapling is stenosis, which seems to occur more often than after a hand-sewn anastomosis. Some studies

suggest that up to 40 per cent of pouches with a stapled anal anastomosis can stenose and therefore require repeated dilatation or the
daily use of anal dilators. In order for the patient to maximize the use
of dilators, it is important that he or she is instructed in the proper
use of either Hegar's or St Mark's dilators (Figure 8.5).

The patient should initially be instructed to empty the pouch to
the best of his or her ability. The dilator should then be lubricated
using lubricating jelly. With the patient lying on the left side, the dilator should be inserted carefully and gently through the anus and into
the pouch. The amount inserted into the pouch depends on the type
of dilator in use. Once inside the pouch, the dilator should be turned
through 360 degrees and then gently removed. Both the anal area
and the dilator should be wiped clean. Once the procedure has been
completed, the patient may need to evacuate the pouch once more.
It is generally recommended that this be repeated once or twice a
day. The general care of the dilator involves washing it in hot soapy
water, drying it thoroughly and storing it somewhere safe.

Both a hand-sewn and a stapled anal anastomosis using an endo-
anal technique can lead to damage to the anal sphincter (Nicholls et
al 1981a, Seow-Choen et al 1991). There is some evidence to show
that, following anal anastomosis, the resting anal tone is reduced and
likely to remain so indefinitely. Efforts are thus made to limit the

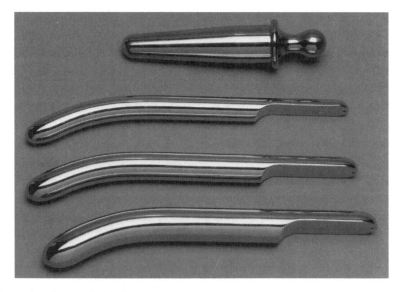

Figure 8.5 Hegars/St Mark's dilators.

degree of trauma to the internal anal sphincter during the surgical procedure (Wexner et al 1989).

The use of anal manometry

Some studies (Sharp et al 1987) have proposed the use of anal manometry as mandatory in the preoperative phase, whereas others (Morgado et al 1994) suggest that it is beneficial only within a research setting. Numerous factors may contribute to the adverse impact upon the internal anal sphincter. It was initially thought that prolonged anal dilatation in the process of rectal mucosectomy was a significant factor (Johnston et al 1987, Primrose et al 1988, Tuckson & Fazio 1991), but subsequent studies involving either a limited mucosectomy or no mucosectomy at all have shown a postoperative fall in resting anal canal tone (Pricolo et al 1996).

Most surgeons choose to transect the rectum very close to the anorectal junction and in doing so almost certainly interfere with nerve endings to the internal anal sphincter, causing the loss of the recto-anal inhibitory reflex. This has been highlighted as being either temporary or permanent (Nicholls et al 1981a).

Other studies have looked into the usefulness of pelvic floor exercises (Jorge et al 1994) (Table 8.2), concluding that sphincter-strengthening exercises before closing the loop ileostomy did not ameliorate the transient impairment of function. It seems that pelvic floor exercises are unlikely to cause harm, but patients who have recently undergone pouch surgery should not be encouraged to undertake the exercises for fear of anastomotic breakdown.

Some early trials have investigated the use of topical phenylephrine as a way to increase anal sphincter resting pressure (Carapeti et al 1999). If it proves successful, this could be a novel therapeutic approach to the treatment of passive faecal incontinence.

Temporary loop ileostomy

The temporary loop ileostomy can prove to be extremely difficult for the patient to manage, not only practically, but also physiologically; thus, controversy has arisen over whether there is a need to defunction the pouch at all.

Many surgeons prefer routinely to use a diverting ileostomy following ileo-anal pouch surgery. This is mainly because of the large

Table 8.2 Pelvic floor exercises

1. Sit, stand or lie with your knees slightly apart. Tighten and pull up the sphincter muscles as tightly as you can. Hold them tight for at least 5 seconds, and then relax for at least 10 seconds. Repeat at least 5 times. This will work on the strength of your muscles
2. Next, pull the muscles up to about half of their maximum squeeze. See how long you can hold this for. Then relax for at least 10 seconds. Repeat at least 5 times. This will work on the endurance or staying power of your muscles
3. Pull up the muscles as quickly and tightly as you can; then relax and then pull them up again. See how many times you can do this before you get tired. Try for at least 5 quick pull-ups
4. Do these exercises – 5 as hard as you can, 5 as long as you can and as many quick pull-ups as you can – at least 10 times a day
5. As the muscles get stronger, you will find that you can hold for longer than 5 seconds and that you can do more pull-ups each time without the muscle getting tired
6. It takes time to make the muscles stronger. You may need to exercise regularly for several months before they gain their full strength

Information from *Sphincter exercises for people with bowel control problems*, St Mark's Hospital Patient Information Series.

number of suture and stapled lines involved in pouch surgery and the fact that many patients with ulcerative colitis are taking steroids and are to some extent malnourished. The consequences of anastomotic leakage and pelvic sepsis are therefore greatly reduced. Several studies have, however, shown that pouch formation without a covering loop ileostomy does not have detrimental consequences on immediate postoperative recovery or in fact the long-term functioning of the pouch (Mowschenson & Critchlow 1995).

The arguments against a defunctioning ileostomy include avoidance of the morbidity associated with the procedure, the reduced cost of another operation and the shorter treatment time. On the other hand, an ileostomy minimizes the consequences of anastomotic leakage and pelvic sepsis should either occur, and it is also very useful for the patient to have experienced an ileostomy. In the event of function being disappointing, the patient at least knows what the alternative is.

Living with a temporary loop ileostomy has been described by many patients, especially those who have experienced an end-ileostomy, as being an extremely traumatic experience. Salter

(1992a) demonstrated that, when comparing feelings towards an alteration in body image between those with permanent ileostomies and those with internal pouches, these were much the same. Employing further exploration, the authors reported that those with an internal pouch maintained vivid memories of life with a temporary loop ileostomy and often feared that if they were ever to lose the pouch, their quality of life would be unbearable.

In practical terms, the temporary loop ileostomy can be difficult for patients to manage. This is generally because of the increased likelihood of stomal retraction and/or mucosal separation (Figure 8.6 and Plate 13), the corrosive nature of the effluent, as a result of its high content of prolytic enzymes, the high stomal output, leading to water and electrolyte imbalance, and mucosal discharge from the distal end of the stoma. These problems are likely to occur in the immediate postoperative period and may prolong the patient's stay in hospital. It is therefore particularly important for the clinical nurse specialist in stoma care to be vigilant in order to decrease management problems and promote comprehensive rehabilitation.

Stomal retraction can cause leakage problems, leading to excoriation of the peristomal skin. There is also a risk of contamination of the pouch as effluent from the proximal loop spills over into the distal loop and consequently down into the pouch. Some ostomy manufacturers now produce appliances with an integrated convexity, thus

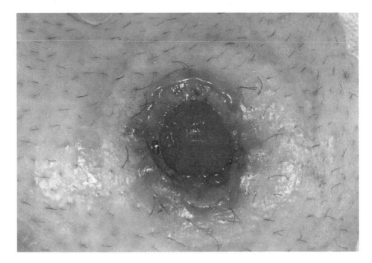

Figure 8.6 Mucosal separation with stomal retraction (see Plate 13).

allowing the proximal loop of the ileostomy to protrude. This will ultimately encourage effluent to fall down into the appliance rather than slipping underneath the base of the appliance, minimizing leakage and the occurrence of excoriated peristomal skin. These appliances can be used in conjunction with a belt in order to obtain a greater depth of convexity.

If mucosal separation has occurred, discussion must take place with the surgeon, treatment aiming for the healing of the separation whilst maintaining skin integrity. A successful treatment used at St Mark's Hospital includes initially removing any loose sutures from within the separation, and irrigating the area with water or saline. The area is then dried with a cool hairdryer. Once it is dry, either Orabase™ paste or Orahesive™ powder is used to fill the cavity created by the separation. A thin hydrocolloid wafer is then placed over the top to act as a seal, and the patient's usual appliance is applied. Convexity within the appliance can prove useful here too. The site needs observing either daily or on alternate days depending on the severity of mucosal separation.

The patient must be made aware that stomal output is likely to be greater and more aggressive in nature than with an end-ileostomy because the distal end of the ileum leading towards the pouch and the pouch itself lie dormant whilst the healing process takes place. Some suggest that the phase during which patients have undergone pouch surgery and have a loop ileostomy can be equated to the case of somebody with short gut syndrome and should therefore be treated in the same manner. The appliance that is normally worn will need to be made more robust to withhold the corrosive stomal output. In most cases, a washer or seal may be used in addition to the normal appliance (Figure 8.7), and it is recommended that the patient change his or her appliance daily if using a one-piece system and on alternate days if using a two-piece device.

Sodium depletion

It is natural to expect the effluent from the temporary loop ileostomy to be excessive in the early postoperative period: some patients experience an output of 2 litres over 24 hours. This may be due to the stoma being placed too proximally, but in most cases a functional cause is presumed. The output usually settles within a week or two.

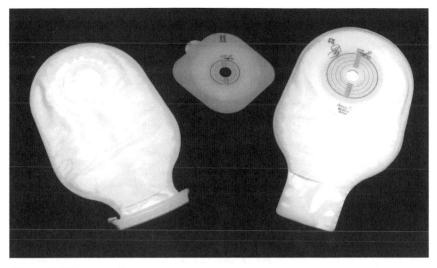

Figure 8.7 Stoma appliances.

Water and sodium loss is a common problem, and it is important that the ileostomy output is measured and the general condition of the patient monitored to anticipate features of sodium depletion, which causes a contraction of the intravascular compartment. Symptoms include weakness, postural hypotension, anorexia, nausea, tachycardia associated with peripheral vasoconstriction, raised urea and electrolyte levels, low urinary output and acidosis (which if severe will lead to renal failure).

In patients currently or recently taking steroids, sodium loss through the kidney may be an additional factor leading to sodium depletion. Adrenocortical suppression as a result of steroid medication, combined with sodium depletion, can precipitate an Addisonian crisis. In such cases, steroids should be given along with an intravenous infusion of normal saline, which should apply to all cases. The patient's progress should be monitored by measuring the ileostomy and urine output and serum electrolyte levels.

The possibility of sodium depletion should be explained to all patients prior to discharge from hospital, and if there is any doubt over the patient's competence to add salt to food, a rehydration solution should be prescribed (Figure 8.8). If the patient is unable to maintain his or her fluid and electrolyte balance, admission may be required for intravenous fluid treatment.

Electrolyte Mix (St Mark's Hospital Formula)

Name   Date

You have been prescribed Electrolyte Mix. You will need to make up the solution fresh each day. You will need to measure out the three ingredients using the three scoops that you have been given: one for each of the three powders. Measure SIX level 5ml spoonsful of Glucose, ONE heaped 2.5ml spoonful of the Sodium Bicarbonate (SOD BIC) and ONE level 5ml spoonful of the Sodium Chloride (SOD CHL) and dissolve in 1 litre of tap water.

Drink .... litre(s) of this mixture throughout the day.

You can buy the powders from any community pharmacy and some supermarkets. Sodium Chloride is table salt, which you will have in your home already. Sodium Bicarbonate is also known as Bicarbonate of Soda. These are cheaper to buy directly than to obtain on prescription if you pay prescription charges.

If you need to get these prescribed, please show your GP this leaflet. They will need to be prescribed in the following way:

R$_x$ St Mark's Electrolyte Mix

Formula:-	Glucose	20g)
	Sodium Chloride	3.5g) made up to 1 litre with
	Sodium Bicarbonate	2.5g) tap water daily
Mitte:-	Glucose powder	....g
	Sodium Chloride powder	....g
	Sodium Bicarbonate powder	....g

If the prescription is written in this way, your community Pharmacist can claim for these items and will be able to supply you.

Figure 8.8 Rehydration mix.

Poor function

As described in Chapter 4, a pouch functions between 3 and 7 times in each 24 hour period. When reporting functional results, it is important to take into consideration the frequency of defaecation per 24 hours, the number of defaecations at night, urgency, mode of evacuation, the need for anti-diarrhoeal medication, continence and the presence of anal skin excoriation. There are several reasons for abnormal frequency, the most important being chronic intestinal obstruction, an evacuation disorder, inflammation of the pouch (pouchitis), a small-capacity pouch and a weak sphincter, some of which have the potential for improvement.

It is important that an accurate assessment of the patient is made, which will include a detailed history, clinical examination and investigations. Taking the patient's history will reveal systemic symptoms more suggestive of intestinal obstruction and pouchitis rather than a local mechanical problem. Digital examination per anum will detect stricture formation. Pouchoscopy will demonstrate a long distal ileal segment and mucosal inflammation. Investigations such as a defaecating pouchogram to identify the effectiveness of pouch emptying, a small bowel barium enema and follow-through to detect obstruction above the pouch and biopsy of the pouch to exclude inflammation can prove useful.

It is known that the function of the pouch improves with time. During the period of adjustment, many patients take anti-diarrhoeal medication. It is quite safe for them to titrate the dose of anti-diarrhoeal medication under the guidance of a health-care professional, and many do this in conjunction with regulating their dietary intake. Many patients need support and reassurance during this period over the use of the medication and dietary choices (see Chapter 9).

Frequency may be an idiosyncratic feature, determined presumably by the intrinsic motility of the intestine in a particular person. This functional frequency is sometimes phasic. For example, the patient may go infrequently whilst at work but once at home go several times in quick succession during the evening or at night. Little can be done apart from re-educating the patient to try to empty the pouch whilst regulating function with anti-diarrhoeal medication.

It is reported night evacuation occurs in 20–50 per cent of patients (Sagar et al 1993). It is probably the most sensitive symptomatic guide to function. Although the need to get up at night gradually ceases with time in most patients, some are still left with troublesome night-time frequency. This may also be associated with night-time leakage and faecal incontinence. Adjusting meal patterns and/or excluding some problematic foods from the diet may help this situation.

Outflow obstruction

In some cases, leakage is caused by incomplete emptying of the pouch, so some patients are advised to use a rectal catheter to aid the emptying (Table 8.3).

Incomplete emptying can result from a stenosis (stricture) or the presence of a significant distal ileal or rectal segment between the pouch and the anus. A distal ileal segment is part of the 'S' design and, if long, may cause outflow obstruction. A rectal segment occurs when the pouch–anal anastomosis is made too high, thus retaining

Table 8.3 Use of the rectal (medina) catheter to aid ileo-anal pouch evacuation

This procedure is undertaken in the toilet (with an accessible hand basin)

1. Prepare the equipment: Medina catheter
                                 Lubricating gel
                                 Toilet tissue
                                 Bladder syringe (optional)

2. Ask the patient to empty their pouch to the best of their ability
3. Guide the patient in locating their anus using the patient's index finger. This may be helped by the patient squatting over the toilet or lifting their right buttock from the toilet seat
4. Ask the patient to lubricate the 'eyelet' end of the medina catheter
5. The patient is then encouraged to insert the lubricated end of the catheter into their pouch via the anus. This is when most patients will feel tense, which may cause the pouch to go into spasm and make insertion difficult. The patient must thus be encouraged to relax
6. The funnelled end of the catheter must be aimed towards the toilet
7. Once the catheter has been correctly inserted into the pouch, the pouch should begin to empty. The patient may pass only wind initially
8. If the pouch effluent begins to empty slowly, the patient should be encouraged to activate the abdominal muscles by coughing or laughing. The abdomen can also be massaged
9. If the pouch effluent is thick in consistency, the patient will need to irrigate the pouch with the aid of a bladder syringe and warm tap water. Warm water can be instilled in volumes of 30–50 ml at a time, depending on what the patient can tolerate, up to a total of 500–1000 ml. The water should only be instilled rather than being drawn back via the syringe
10. The pouch sometimes empties completely and causes suction in the pouch, or the eyelets of the catheter may become lodged at the pouch–anal anastomosis. If this occurs, the patient should again try to relax. A small amount of air or water can be inserted into the pouch via the bladder syringe in order to release the catheter

rectal mucosa. Surgical salvage to rectify the problem is feasible. In the case of stenosis, dilatation is performed either in the outpatient department or under general anaesthetic, depending on severity.

In some cases, there appears to be no physiological reason, other than that the ability to defaecate is different, why pouch function is poor. Normal defaecation results from the contraction and relaxation of both smooth and striated muscle within the colon and rectum. The pouch patient, however, effectively lacks the ability to contract and relax 'new' muscles, and in some cases find biofeedback therapy is useful. In this patients are educated and re-trained in the mechanics of defaecation.

Drugs

There is a concern that some medications will not be absorbed within the small intestine. These include drugs that are enteric coated and/or modified-release, that is, slow-release, tablets. In these instances, advice from a doctor or pharmacist should be sought prior to administration.

Many female patients are concerned about family planning and taking the contraceptive pill. Most contraceptive pills are absorbed within the duodenum, so patients should be able to absorb the drug as effectively as those with an ileostomy. There is also evidence to suggest that female patients are able to absorb the 'morning after pill' (Guillebaud 1993). When advising patients on family planning, it should, however, be recommended that both partners use some form of contraception.

Diet

Patients are often concerned about what they should and should not eat or drink, usually learning by trial and error what will provide them with satisfactory pouch function. There is evidence to suggest that many pouch patients modify their dietary intake to suit their new lifestyle. Many avoid certain foods, whereas others will change their meal pattern (Bond et al 1997). Research into exclusion diets in pouch patients is being undertaken at the John Radcliffe Hospital, Oxford. Foods suggested to increase and decrease pouch function are highlighted in Table 8.4, and these issues are discussed in more depth in Chapter 9.

Table 8.4 Food affecting pouch function

Foods that thicken the stools	Foods that loosen the stools
Bananas	Chocolate
Rice	Raw fruits
Bread	Raw vegetables
Potatoes	Highly spiced foods
Creamy peanut butter	Fried foods
Marshmallows	Greasy foods
Cheese	Sugary foods
Tapioca	Fruit juice (grape or prune)
Yoghurt	Leafy green vegetables
Pasta	
Pretzels	

Despite the known high complication rate of pouch surgery, patients remain keen to undergo this procedure. Several quality of life (Bond et al 1997, Seidel et al 1999, Tiainen & Matikainen 1999) studies indicate that patients prefer to adjust their lifestyle in whatever manner necessary in order to remain ileostomy-free. A satisfactory outcome of surgery has been identified in 87 per cent of patients (Belliveau et al 1999).

Considering all these controversies and difficulties surrounding the ileo-anal pouch, what does its future hold? Surgeons will always show a personal preference for a particular surgical technique and pouch management, whether it is a 'J' or 'W' shaped pouch, or a hand-sewn versus stapled anastomosis, or the latest treatment for pouchitis. Our knowledge is enhanced through objective clinical studies, and, as health-care professionals, we should be aiming to learn about the long-term changes within pouch care, including new treatments for pouchitis, anal sphincter function and other specific complications.

In order to optimize the benefits of the pouch procedure, it is important that both the patient and the multidisciplinary professionals involved in care understand the various aspects of fine-tuning pouch function, including diet, medication and lifestyle. In managing pouch dysfunction, the temptation to delay treatment and advice should be resisted; instead, an approach that is systematic and understanding should be adopted (Thompson-Fawcett et al 1997).

CHAPTER 9

Dietary aspects of internal pouches

MORAG PEARSON

Diet plays an important role in the management of people with internal pouches. As pouches are formed from terminal ileum after colonic resection, this has implications for the absorption of fluid, electrolytes and nutrients, and in turn for the maintenance of an adequate nutritional status. In addition, the nutritional status of people approaching pouch surgery depends on their general health and underlying condition. Some will require nutritional support preoperatively, and all will need guidance and support with the re-introduction of food postoperatively.

People with established pouches can manage a varied and healthy diet. Although most find their stool frequency acceptable, some, however, empirically associate changes in pouch function with variations in diet and may restrict their diet to control pouch function. There are few published data on the relationship between diet and pouch function to support dietary recommendations.

This chapter considers the nutritional implications of internal pouch formation and summarises current dietary advice for people with both new and established pouches. It focuses mainly on ileo-anal pouches but indicates where there are differences for Kock pouches.

Nutritional implications of internal pouch formation

Understanding the effect of pouch formation on water, sodium and nutrient absorption will enable the reader to grasp potential nutritional problems and the principles of dietary advice. This section describes absorption in the normal gut and the changes that occur after internal pouch formation.

Absorption of water, sodium and nutrients in the normal gut

Each day, food and beverages, plus 3.5–5.0 litres of fluid comprising saliva, gastric and pancreatic secretions and bile, enter the jejunum. The jejunum, ileum and colon differ markedly in the way in which they absorb water and sodium (Figure 9.1).

Absorption of nutrients   **Absorption of water and sodium**

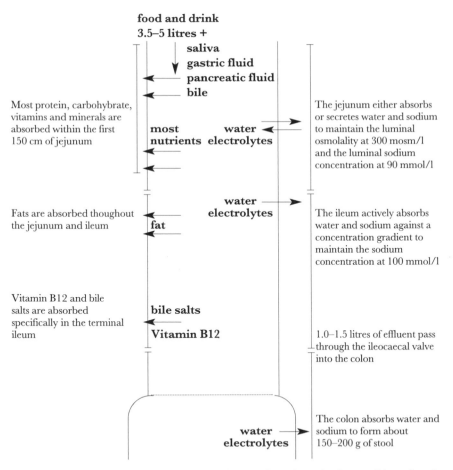

food and drink
3.5–5 litres +
saliva
gastric fluid
pancreatic fluid
bile

Most protein, carbohybrate, vitamins and minerals are absorbed within the first 150 cm of jejunum

most nutrients   **water electrolytes**

The jejunum either absorbs or secretes water and sodium to maintain the luminal osmolality at 300 mosm/l and the luminal sodium concentration at 90 mmol/l

water electrolytes

Fats are absorbed thoughout the jejunum and ileum

fat

The ileum actively absorbs water and sodium against a concentration gradient to maintain the sodium concentration at 100 mmol/l

Vitamin B12 and bile salts are absorbed specifically in the terminal ileum

bile salts

Vitamin B12

1.0–1.5 litres of effluent pass through the ileocaecal valve into the colon

water electrolytes

The colon absorbs water and sodium to form about 150–200 g of stool

Figure 9.1 The absorption of water, sodium and nutrients in the small bowel and colon. Adapted from Lennard-Jones (1991).

In the jejunum, water and sodium are either absorbed from or secreted into the lumen to maintain the osmolarity of the intraluminal contents at 300 mosm/l and the sodium concentration at 90 mmol/l. Sodium absorption is also linked to the absorption of nutrients, in particular glucose. In contrast, in the ileum, water and sodium are absorbed, with the absorption of sodium taking place against a concentration gradient and without any linkage to glucose. This reduces the effluent volume passing through the ileocaecal valve to about 1000 ml containing approximately 100 mmol sodium. The colon readily absorbs both water and sodium to produce about 100–150 g stool, which contains very little sodium (Lennard-Jones 1994).

Most nutrients, including protein, carbohydrates, vitamins and minerals, are absorbed in the first 200 cm of the jejunum. Fat is absorbed throughout the jejunum and ileum, whereas bile acids and vitamin B12 are absorbed specifically in the terminal ileum (Lennard-Jones 1994).

Effect of internal pouch formation on gut physiology

Proctocolectomy results in a loss of the colon and its function of absorbing water and sodium. The pouch itself is formed from 30–60 cm of terminal ileum, which is the specific site for the absorption of bile acids and vitamin B12, and which subsequently adopts the new role of faecal reservoir to reduce bowel frequency.

Over time, the ileal mucosa of the pouch changes to a more colonic type mucosa with partial villous atrophy, chronic inflammation, crypt hyperplasia and colonic metaplasia (Go et al 1987, Bain et al 1995). The microflora of the pouch increases to become intermediate between that of ileostomy effluent and that of normal faeces, with implications for the bacterial degradation of bile acids and vitamin B12 (Brandberg et al 1972, Nasmyth & Williams 1993).

Most people with an internal pouch demonstrate good health, maintaining or increasing their body weight (Chartrand-Lefebvre et al 1990, Öjerskog et al 1990) and rarely developing clinical signs of malabsorption or malnutrition (Lerch et al 1989). Studies of the effect of internal pouch formation on nutrient absorption have focused mainly on water, sodium, bile acids and vitamin B12.

Water and sodium absorption after internal pouch formation

People with an ileo-anal pouch open their pouch on average 3–7 times a day, passing a daily average of 650 g of stool of a semi-solid, mushy or liquid consistency (Nicholls et al 1981b, Pemberton 1993). Those with a Kock pouch intubate 2–4 times per day, passing a daily average of 740 g of stool (Brevinge et al 1992a). Their daily faecal weight, urinary volume and urinary excretion of sodium are similar to those of people with conventional ileostomies (Santavirta et al 1991, Brevinge et al 1992b).

Both groups maintain normal body stores of water and salt by compensating for the higher faecal losses through the renal conservation of water and sodium (Christie et al 1990). This compensatory mechanism increases the incidence of renal calculi in both groups (Stern et al 1980, Christie et al 1996). Some of the lost colonic function may also be compensated for by an increased absorption of water and salt in the ileum (Lerch et al 1989).

Bile acid absorption after internal pouch formation

Several studies have demonstrated a malabsorption of bile acids after pouch formation (Nilsson et al 1979, Hylander et al 1986, Fiorentini et al 1987, Lerch et al 1989, Salemans et al 1993, Bain et al 1995), but it is not clear whether this is caused by a dysfunction in active mucosal transport or by a bacterial degradation of bile acids that reduces their availability for reabsorption.

The loss of this enterohepatic circulation could reduce the bile acid pool, leading to fat malabsorption and an increased risk of gallstone formation (Nasmyth & Williams 1993, Salemans & Nagengast 1995). Fat malabsorption has been documented in some studies (Nilsson et al 1979, Fiorentini et al 1987, M'Koma 1994), whereas others have noted normal fat absorption (Nicholls et al 1981b, Heppel et al 1982, Hylander et al 1986). There is to date no documented evidence that people with an internal pouch have an increased incidence of cholelithiasis (Öjerskog et al 1990, Harvey et al 1991).

Vitamin B12 absorption after internal pouch formation

In a study of 83 people 3 years after ileo-anal pouch formation, 11 per cent had a low serum vitamin B12 level and 36 per cent showed impaired B12 absorption, as indicated by a low Schilling test result

(M'Koma 1994b). Similar results have been demonstrated by other studies (Jagenburg et al 1975, Nicholls et al 1981b, Nilsson et al 1984, Hojlund Pederson et al 1985, O'Connell et al 1986, Fiorentini et al 1987, Hylander et al 1991). It is again not clear whether this deficiency is caused by an inadequate intake, a dysfunction of mucosal transport across the terminal ileum or the bacterial binding of vitamin B12 in the pouch, rendering it unavailable for absorption (Nasmyth et al 1993, M'Koma 1994b).

Absorption of other nutrients after internal pouch formation

Three studies have noted a reduction in the absorption of carbohydrate and protein after ileo-anal pouch formation, raising the question of whether there is a loss of small bowel function following the adaptive changes within the ileal mucosa (Fiorentini et al 1987, Lerch et al 1989, Stelzner et al 1990).

Serum folate levels were normal, but a minority of people with an ileo-anal pouch were found to have a low haemoglobin level or low serum iron level (Nicholls et al 1981b, Lerch et al 1989, M'Koma 1994b). It is unclear whether these were caused by inadequate intake, impaired absorption, increased requirements or blood loss (M'Koma 1994b).

Further research is clearly required with regard to the food intake, nutrient absorption and nutritional status of people with internal pouches. Meanwhile, it is important to encourage them to take a balanced diet to help prevent nutrient deficiencies and to monitor their fluid balance, weight, iron and vitamin B12 status and any clinical signs of deficiency at outpatient follow-up.

Dietary advice for patients with a loop ileostomy or new internal pouch

Nursing staff play a central role in identifying and supporting patients at risk of malnutrition or dehydration (Table 9.1) and in guiding them with food re-introduction postoperatively (Table 9.2).

Nutritional support

Prior to pouch surgery, patients may present with varying degrees of malnutrition depending on their general health and underlying condition. Those with ulcerative colitis are especially at risk because

Table 9.1: The role of nursing staff in the dietary management of patients with internal pouches

Role	Process	Action
• Identify patients who are malnourished	• Check weight and use a nutrition screening tool for all new admissions • Liaise with doctors, dietitians and stoma care nurses to develop local protocols for nutrition screening, the monitoring of nutritional status and the management of malnourished patients • Identify training needs and arrange training for nursing and support staff	• Refer malnourished patients to the dietitian for nutritional assessment and advice
• Identify patients who are at risk of becoming malnourished	• As above	• Document the problem • Explain the importance of eating and drinking to patients and assist them with menu, snack and enriched food choices • Monitor their food intake and regularly re-check their weight and nutrition score. If their nutrition score deteriorates, refer them to the dietitian
• Identify patients who are at risk of becoming dehydrated	• Monitor weight, fluid intake and urine and stool output, and observe for any signs of dehydration or sodium depletion • Liaise with doctors, dietitians and stoma care nurses to local protocols for managing high outputs and fluid develop balance Identify training needs and arrange training for nursing and support staff	• Document the problem and liaise with the doctors and stoma care nurses over management • Educate patients on the importance of taking electrolyte solution and restricting non-electroyte fluids. Assist them with menu choices • Provide anti-diarrhoeal agents 30–60 minutes before food • Monitor fluid balance and inform the doctor of any deterioration
• Guide patients on the re-introduction of food postoperatively	• Liaise with doctors, dietitians and stoma care nurses to develop local protocols for the re-introduction of fluid and food postoperatively • Identify training needs and arrange training for nursing and support staff	• Explain the process of fluid and food re-introduction postoperatively and help the patient with menu choices • Provide support and monitor food intake • Refer any patient with problems to the dietitian
• Guide patients with setablished pouches to choose a healthy diet	• Liaise with dietitians and stoma care nurses to agree healthy eating guidelines • Identify training needs and arrange training for nursing and support staff	• Explain the importance of healthy eating, and guide patients using the locally agreed education tool • Note any patient who is underweight or has a restricted eating pattern and refer to the dietitian

Table 9.2 Dietary advice for people with new stomas or internal pouches

- Introduce a soft, low-fibre diet to avoid blockages or any disturbance of the surgical wound during healing
- Choose a high-protein and high-energy diet to promote healing and prevent weight loss
- Overcome poor appetite by taking small, frequent meals or snacks and including energy-dense foods
- Take commercial sip-feeds between meals if the appetite is very poor
- After 2–4 weeks, re-introduce fibrous foods in small quantities, to be chewed well

both acute and chronic disease are associated with factors such as reduced food intake, increased intestinal losses and increased nutritional requirements.

Patients with active ulcerative colitis experience anorexia and may reduce their food intake to minimize symptoms such as nausea, pain or diarrhoea. Anxiety, depression and drug side-effects can further intensify this anorexia. Blood and protein are lost from inflamed bowel, and fluid and electrolytes through diarrhoea, yet nutritional requirements are increased by inflammation, fever and surgery. Malnutrition can delay recovery, slow wound healing, increase susceptibility to infection, reduce stamina and lower mood.

Preoperative nutritional care should ideally be considered when elective surgery is planned, but nursing staff should screen all new admissions, by checking their weight and using a nutrition score or other simple screening tool, to identify those who are malnourished and those who are nutritionally at risk (Bond 1997). Malnourished patients should be referred to the dietitian for nutritional assessment and advice. Nursing staff can help nutritionally at-risk patients to maximize their food intake by guiding their menu choice and suggesting that those with a poor appetite take smaller meals, supplemented with snacks in between.

Meals should include a portion of protein (meat, fish, cheese, eggs, milk, yoghurt or pulses) for tissue repair and a portion of starchy carbohydrate (bread, cereal, potato, rice or pasta) for energy. Nutritious puddings include milk puddings, custard, blancmanges, yoghurt or cheese and biscuits. Nutritious snacks include sandwiches, cereal, milky drinks or cold puddings, which can be saved and eaten 1–2 hours after the main meal. Patients may also supplement their main meals with energy-dense foods such as butter, margarine, cream, sugar, jam, honey, marmalade, sweets, chocolates, biscuits, cakes, ice cream and crisps.

Those with a very poor intake may benefit from a commercial sip-feed to increase their energy and nutrient intake. Depending on local policy, this may be given by nursing staff or prescribed by the dietitian or doctor. Patients should be encouraged to take sip-feeds in between meals and to try alternatives if at first they are unacceptable. Nursing staff should monitor patients' food intake and re-check their weight and nutrition score regularly so that any who deteriorate can be identified and referred to the dietitian.

Re-introducting food after surgery

Intravenous fluids are given postoperatively until the bowel sounds return and flatus is passed from the stoma or pouch. Patients may then introduce fluids, followed by a soft, low-fibre diet.

Fibrous foods such as nuts, seeds, pips, pith, fruit or vegetable skins, raw vegetables, peas, sweetcorn, mushroom, dried fruit, coconut and pineapple have the potential to cause a blockage because they resist digestion. If fibrous foods are eaten in large quantities or are not properly chewed, they may form a food plug that can stick at the point where the ileum narrows as it passes through the abdominal wall to form the stoma, or at the ileostomy closure site, especially if tissue is swollen postoperatively. Fibrous foods can also block the drainage catheter used to empty a Kock pouch (Beart 1979, cited in Cranley 1983).

Patients with a new stoma or ileo-anal pouch are therefore advised to follow a low-fibre diet for 2–4 weeks after surgery. Thereafter, they may re-introduce fibrous foods in small quantities, making sure that they are properly chewed. They may initially wish to be cautious with those foods more frequently reported to upset pouch function (Table 9.3).

Patients with a Kock pouch are advised to introduce a puréed or soft low-fibre diet for first 2 weeks while the reservoir catheter is in situ. Thereafter, they may switch to a low-fibre diet provided that the food is thoroughly chewed, adopting a normal diet after 4 weeks provided they take care with fibrous foods (see Chapter 5). Should patients experience a blockage, they are advised to stop food but

Table 9.3 Food and associated symptoms reported by people with internal pouches

Symptoms	Associated foods
Increased stool output	Fibrous foods, for example pulses, leafy green vegetables, raw vegetables, raw fruits, wholegrain cereals, nuts, sweetcorn, spicy foods, alcohol, caffeinated beverages, fruit juices, fried foods, chocolate and milk
Decreased stool output	Bread, rice, pasta and bananas
Anal irritation	Spicy foods, nuts, seeds, coconut, citrus fruits and juices, raw fruit and vegetables
Increased wind	Broccoli, sprouts, cabbage, cauliflower, onion, garlic, leeks, asparagus, beans, spicy foods, beer, milk, fizzy drinks
Increased stool odour	Fish, onions, garlic, eggs

Data from Lerch et al 1989, Wexner et al 1989, Chartrand-Lefebvre et al 1990, Fujita et al 1992, Tyus et al 1992 and unpublished surveys by the Kangaroo Group (1994) and Red Lion Group (1997).

continue sipping fluids and contact their doctor or stoma care nurse. Patients should be encouraged to develop a regular eating pattern to help to establish an acceptable stoma or pouch function.

High output from stoma or pouch

In the early postoperative phase, both stoma and new pouch patients may experience high-volume liquid stools of greater than 1 litre over 24 hours. This may be caused by the stoma being placed too proximally in the ileum or by a temporary functional disorder that settles with time (Nicholls 1993). It may cause the patient to become dehydrated and sodium depleted, so nursing staff need to keep strict fluid balance records and watch for signs of depletion (Table 9.4).

Dehydration is indicated by a urine volume of less than 1 litre in 24 hours and sodium depletion by a random urinary concentration of less than 20 mmol of sodium per litre. Because of the influence of the renin-angiotensin mechanism, the plasma sodium concentration remains normal until the body stores are severely depleted. Physical signs become apparent before major changes in blood chemistry and include thirst, lethargy, cramps, sunken dark-ringed eyes, reduced skin turgor, a rapid low-volume pulse, dizziness on standing as a

Table 9.4 Assessment of high output from stoma or internal pouch

- Fluid balance records (24 hour fluid intake, stoma or pouch output and urine output)
- Daily body weight
- Blood pressure when lying and standing
- Blood urea and serum electrolyte levels
- Random urine sodium concentration
- Clinical signs of sodium depletion

result of postural hypotension and rapidly decreasing body weight (1 kg being equivalent to 1 litre of fluid) (Wood 1996).

In response to the thirst, the patient will drink water or other hypotonic fluids, which dilute the jejunal sodium concentration to below 90 mmol/l and cause sodium to be secreted into the luminal fluid to raise its concentration back to 90 mmol/l. When the ileostomy or pouch output is high, much of this sodium-enriched effluent is lost, increasing the patient's thirst and perpetuating the cycle.

The remedy is to reduce the jejunal secretion of sodium by restricting the patient's intake of hypotonic fluids to 1 litre and meeting fluid requirements with a glucose–electrolyte solution, which will promote absorption in the jejunum. A modification of the World Health Organization's oral rehydration solution, which contains 90 mmol of sodium per litre, is suitable (20 g of glucose, 3.5 g of sodium chloride and 2.5 g of sodium bicarbonate or citrate added to 1 litre of tap water). This tastes like sweet salt water, and its palatability can be improved by chilling it and flavouring it with a small amount of squash or fruit juice. Patients should sip 1 litre of this electrolyte mix throughout the day.

An anti-diarrhoeal agent such as loperamide or codeine phosphate will help to thicken the stool and reduce output. This should be taken 30–45 minutes before food and at bed-time, in increasing doses until control is achieved. Other helpful measures include continuing the low-fibre diet and taking fluid separately from meals in order to slow transit, promote absorption and reduce intestinal losses (Wood 1996) (Table 9.5).

At this stage, it may be difficult to motivate patients to eat and drink because they may be afraid that this will increase their

Table 9.5 Management of a high output from a stoma or internal pouch

- If severely sodium depleted, administer 0.9 per cent sodium chloride intravenously until the urinary sodium concentration is greater than 20 mmol/l
- Take 1 litre of electrolyte mix (90 mmol sodium/l) sipped throughout the day
- Restrict non-electrolyte fluids to 1 litre
- Take anti-diarrhoeal drugs 30–45 minutes before meals and at bed-time
- Eat a low-fibre diet
- Take fluids separately from meals
- Add salt to food

frequency. In fact, the opposite is true, and re-introducing food will help to thicken and slow the output. Starchy carbohydrate foods such as bread, rice and pasta are particularly helpful in doing this. Patients will need much reassurance and encouragement during this stage until their output begins to settle.

Healthy eating advice for people with established internal pouches

Once the pouch adapts and people become familiar with its usual function, they will feel more confident to experiment with food. Many find that they can enjoy the freedom of a normal unrestricted diet (Table 9.6). Nutrient deficiencies can be avoided by encouraging people to take a varied and balanced diet in line with healthy eating guidelines for the general population. The Health Education Authority's *Balance of Good Health* (Health Education Authority 1996) provides a pictorial guide to achieving a balanced intake from each of the food groups (Figure 9.2).

Protein is essential for the health and repair of body tissues and is found in meat, fish, eggs, pulses, nuts and meat alternatives such as textured vegetable protein, quorn and tofu. People should choose 2–3 portions from this list each day. Red meats, liver, kidney, oily fish, eggs and pulses are good sources of iron and should be regularly included.

Milk, cheese and yoghurt are good sources of calcium, which is important for healthy bones. These foods also provide protein and vitamins. Most people should drink between a half and one pint (300–600 ml) of milk each day or its equivalent as cheese and yoghurt. One cup of milk (200 ml) contains the same amount of

Table 9.6 Dietary advice for people with established pouches

- Eat a varied and well-balanced diet for good health
- Ensure an adequate fluid and salt intake to prevent dehydration
- Develop a regular eating pattern for acceptable pouch function
- Try all foods and only avoid those which repeatedly cause unacceptable symptoms

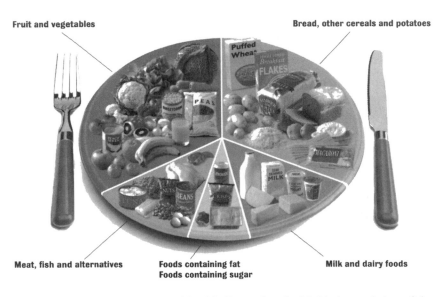

Fruit and vegetables   Bread, other cereals and potatoes

Meat, fish and alternatives   Foods containing fat   Milk and dairy foods
                          Foods containing sugar

Figure 9.2 The balance of good health. Reproduced with kind permission of the Health Education Authority.

calcium as one small carton of yoghurt (120 ml) or 30 g of cheese. Once a healthy weight has been achieved, low-fat alternatives should be encouraged.

Starchy foods provide energy, vitamins and fibre. This group includes bread, chapattis, breakfast cereals, pasta, rice, potatoes, plantains, green bananas and dishes made with cornmeal. These foods are reported to help to thicken the stool and to reduce pouch frequency, so people should choose a variety of foods from this group, making them the main part of their meal and including high-fibre varieties if tolerated.

Fruit and vegetables provide a range of vitamins and minerals, which are essential for good health. Encourage people to choose a variety of foods from this group, aiming for five portions a day. If fruit and vegetables are not well tolerated, peeled fruits, tinned fruits in natural juice, stewed, baked or puréed fruits, unsweetened fruit juices, well-cooked or pureed vegetables and vegetables cooked in soup should be tried instead.

Fats and oils provide energy, essential fats and some vitamins, but too much fat is detrimental to health, so once a healthy weight has been achieved, high-fat foods, including butter, margarine, low-fat spreads, cooking oils, mayonnaise and oily salad dressings, should taken in only small quantities. Foods containing fats and sugars, such as cakes, biscuits, puddings, ice cream, chocolate, sweets, crisps, sugar and sweetened drinks, may be enjoyed as a treat, but they should be taken in small portions and not eaten too often.

In normal circumstances, most people with an internal pouch need 1.5–2.0 litres of **fluid** (8–10 cups of water, tea, coffee, unsweetened fruit juice or sugar-free squashes) and a little extra salt (between a half and one level teaspoon spread throughout the day) to replace losses and prevent dehydration. If fluid loss increases because of an increased output from the pouch, internal pouch owners should take extra salt rather than extra fluid to prevent dehydration. If the symptoms are severe or prolonged, the doctor should be consulted and an electrolyte solution may be prescribed.

An excessive amount of **alcohol** is not good for health. Some types, such as beer or wine, may increase wind and pouch frequency. Alcohol should be taken in moderation, up to a maximum of 3–4 units a day for men and 2–3 units a day for women, with one or two alcohol-free days each week. (It should be noted that 1 unit of alcohol is equal to half a pint of beer, a single measure of spirits, a small glass of sherry or a small glass of wine.)

The relationship between eating pattern, individual foods and pouch function

People with internal pouches associate changes in pouch function with variations in diet, but there are few documented data to support dietary recommendations for this group. Studies of the relationship between eating pattern, individual foods and pouch function have relied on questionnaires, which are very subjective as it may be difficult for pouch owners to identify accurately the effect of specific foods when they are eaten as part of a mixed diet.

Patient perceptions are, however, important as modifiers of eating habits. The studies available found that most people are satisfied with their diet after internal pouch formation, reporting no difficulty in choosing a varied diet, but they do relate eating pattern and individual foods to pouch function (Goldberg 1987, Lerch et al 1989, Wexner et al 1989, Chartrand-Lefebvre et al 1990, Tyus et al 1992, Fujita et al 1992).

In a study of 69 people at least 1 year post-ileostomy closure, the majority opened their pouch 5–8 times per day and between a half and 4 hours after a meal (Tyus et al 1992). Pouch frequency increased with the number of meals eaten, and stool output increased after the largest meal of the day. The authors concluded that people concerned with pouch output should:

- consume no more than three meals a day;
- experiment with the timing and size of their evening meal to reduce pouch frequency at night, for example eating their last meal at least 2 hours before bed-time or switching their largest meal to midday and taking a smaller meal in the evening;
- evaluate their meal and pouch pattern by keeping a diary to determine how long after a meal they could travel.

Studies of the relationship between individual foods and pouch function found that up to one-third of people associated symptoms with specific foods (Goldberg 1987, Chartrand-Lefebvre et al 1990, Fujita 1992, Tyus et al 1992) but that food intolerances were highly variable between people. Rather than suggesting a stringent diet, it is helpful to give people with an internal pouch general guidelines about possible food intolerances (see Table 9.3 above) and encourage them to plan food choices around their own individual tolerance. They should be encouraged to try all foods and avoid only those which repeatedly cause unacceptable pouch function. Tolerance may change with time, so any problem foods should be periodically retried. If people report a number of problem foods, they should be referred to the dietitian to check the nutritional adequacy of their diet.

The effect of fibre seems to vary between people, some finding it beneficial and others finding that it adversely affects pouch function (Wexner et al 1989). Insoluble fibre (in wholemeal bread, wholegrain cereals, fruits and vegetables) has water-holding and stool-bulking properties that may help thicken the stool, but if taken in large quantities they may also cause a faster transit time (Raymond & Becker 1986, Faller et al 1986). Soluble fibre (in oats, pulses, fruit and vegetables) absorbs fluid to form a viscous gel that delays gastric emptying and may slow and thicken the stool output (Wendland 1996). However, not all sources are well tolerated. Internal pouch owners should be encouraged to experiment with fibre to find out which type and what quantity suits them best. Kock pouch owners should avoid or take care to chew thoroughly those fibrous foods which resist digestion and have the potential to block the drainage catheter, for example nuts, seeds, pith, fruit or vegetable skins, raw vegetables, peas, sweetcorn, mushrooms, dried fruit, coconut and pineapple (see Chapter 5).

Wind causes discomfort for some internal pouch owners. It is produced during digestion from swallowed air or from the bacterial fermentation of fibrous food residues in the pouch. It can be lessened by encouraging people to eat regular meals and to avoid eating too much at any one time. Swallowed air may be reduced by eating slowly, chewing the food well, avoiding talking whilst eating and avoiding gum-chewing, mouth-breathing, smoking and taking drinks through a straw. The gas in fizzy drinks may be reduced by pouring the drink into a glass, stirring and leaving it to stand for 10 minutes before drinking. Foods that increase bacterial fermentation are listed in Table 9.3 above, and moderating the quantity eaten may alleviate wind production.

More research is needed to document dietary intake and the relationship between eating pattern, individual foods and pouch function before definitive guidelines can be produced. In the meantime, it is important to encourage internal pouch owners to take a varied and well-balanced diet for good health and, above all, to enjoy their food.

CHAPTER 10

Sexual aspects of internal pouch surgery

MAVE SALTER

The ileo-anal pouch, first described in 1978 by Parks and Nicholls, has been a major advance in the treatment of patients with ulcerative colitis and familial adenomatous polyposis (FAP), as proctocolectomy with restorative intent avoids permanent ileostomy. Over the past 20 years, a large number of these operations have been performed world wide and there have been significant improvements. The great majority of patients now achieve a good result, although the operation unfortunately occasionally fails, and a permanent ileostomy is required (Maxwell, undated). It is, however, important to bear in mind that none of the surgical options will restore the normal, healthy function of the colon and rectum. Therefore an ileo-anal reservoir is not a perfect solution but instead a good alternative in selected patients (Rolstad & Rothenberger, undated).

For the patient with a continent pouch, there may be no visible sign of altered body image from the scar of the suture line (although where a temporary ileostomy has been raised, a small scar is visible on closure). However, the fact that the person has undergone physiological changes in the construction of the ileo-anal pouch, together with its daily activity, may constitute a body image alteration. In terms of sexuality, because of the surgery and resulting physiological changes that the person with an internal pouch undergoes, he or she may feel less attractive and less able to perform sexually.

Beitz (1999) studied the lived experience of 10 patients with an ileo-anal reservoir. Alienation from the body appeared as one category; respondents discussed their feelings of being different, a 'freak'.

Decreased self-respect and confidence were also noted. Role and relationship changes highlighted feelings of inadequate spousal relationships and altered intimacy and gender roles.

When a stoma is raised, an immense price is paid for cure, in terms of both the physical and the psychological impact (Devlin et al 1971). Indeed, Dudley (1978) suggests that however managed, however we delude ourselves, a permanent stoma is an affront, difficult to bear, so that he marvels that professionals and patients have put up with it for so long. To this end, alternatives to conventional stomas have been available for many years (Church 1986). One of the main disadvantages of a stoma is the need to wear an external appliance, and a profound change in body image and sexuality may result from such surgery (Oresland 1996).

It is the aim of this chapter to discuss the nurse's role and the importance of good quality support for the person undergoing an altered body image and perhaps altered sexuality as a result of pouch surgery. It is important to bear in mind that there may already have been body image and sexuality changes resulting from the condition causing the need for surgery (for example, ulcerative colitis) and from a temporary stoma if it was necessary to raise one. Individuals undergoing treatment for a disease often face distressing alterations to their body structure and function, with resulting sexuality changes. Depending on the body part affected and the extent and implications of any physical alterations, patients may experience various degrees of body image concern. This can affect how they feel about themselves and their loved ones and can ultimately influence patients' quality of life (Batchelor et al 1991).

The catastrophic effects of a patient's altered body image on sexuality are often not be taken into account by health-care professionals as body image changes are deemed to be unavoidable and secondary in importance to medical treatment (Guerrero 1997). Similarly, a mind/body duality is perceived to be powerfully maintained in mainstream medicine, which may treat patients with minimal reference to psychology or sociology (Turner 1992). This may lead to a sense of a lack of wholeness which may help to explain the apparent fragility of body image (Rafferty 1995). It is therefore important for the nurse to assess the meaning of sexuality or body image change for individual patients and explore with them interventions for coping (Batchelor et al 1991). Because sexuality and altered body image are so intertwined, it is important to consider both in the nursing care of the patient.

Body image

Body image relates to how we see ourselves and how we feel we appear to others. The unity of body image arises through the influence of the family and results from a dynamic process that develops and changes throughout life (Schilder 1935). Body image is the root of identity, self-esteem and self-worth, the bases from which a person functions. If people are happy with their physical aspects (body image or physical appearance), they are more likely to experience positive feelings of self-esteem (Wassner 1982). In contrast, a person who is unhappy with his physical appearance could have negative feelings regarding him or herself (Burnard & Morrison 1990).

Self-esteem is related to the sense of personal value through acceptance and validation as a sexually desirable person (MacElveen-Hoehn 1985). People who are deformed or disfigured by surgery or other treatment modalities may lose regard for themselves if they feel that important others and society at large do not accept how they look, or they may also feel different because of the altered function of their body (Salter 1997).

Other factors affecting body image formation and dynamics include genetic influences, socialization, fashion, culture, race, education and the mass media (Darbyshire 1986). It is important for nurses to be aware of the social and historical influences that impact on body meaning and thereby influence body image formation and the response to threats against body integrity (Rafferty 1995). In this way, society places great value on having an attractive physical appearance. It influences how a person is perceived by others and valued by them, and how people value themselves.

We are bombarded daily with images of what constitutes the perfect body (Hughes 1991). Because of society's views on physical appearance, the ideal body image has been said to represent youth, beauty, vigour, intactness and health; there is likely to be insecurity and anxiety, and decreased self-esteem, among those who deviate significantly from this ideal (Smitherman 1981). Indeed, those with an ileo-anal pouch may feel less intact than they did previously as a result of the surgery that renders them 'different' because of their need to empty the pouch at more frequent intervals than other people who still have an intact rectum would have their bowels open.

Body image includes the space surrounding the body as well as the accessibility to that space (Horowitz 1966), clothes, make-up and jewellery, as well as aids and accessories, being integrated into body image (Cohen 1991). This may impact on patients with an ileo-anal pouch post-surgery, when they may have attachments such as a naso-gastric tube, drains and an intravenous infusion in place.

Body image changes in the younger person

Children and young adolescents' judgements of their attractiveness are highly predictive of the global self-worth they see in themselves as people (Harter 1982). The importance of appearance is becoming apparent at an increasingly younger age. During adolescence, there is a structural, psychological shift in the individual's identity from being bound up with that of the parent to becoming an 'I' (Kuyk-endall 1988). Illness, for example, inflammatory bowel disease, and the potential need for surgery impinges on this, and an adolescent who has been fighting for independence may be forced back into a dependent role, leading to aggression or depression.

The ego identity shift and struggle to become independent are, however, too threatening to undertake alone, so adolescents unconsciously choose to go through the process in the same way as others in their peer group. They change together; the individual becomes a collective 'I' in the realm of food and clothes, for example, so adolescents requiring surgery may well see themselves as different from their peers. Illness therefore forces the person from the group. It is thus of paramount importance for adolescents undergoing pouch surgery to maintain contact with their friends at this difficult time in their life. If the pouch surgery is undertaken in stages and the patient is well enough, he or she should be encouraged to return to school or college whilst awaiting the next stage of surgery.

Stigma

Goffman (1963) suggests that stigma is the situation of an individual who is disqualified from full social acceptance; a person who has a failing or handicap is reduced in the mind of society as a tainted person. When a person's handicap is not immediately apparent (as in the case of a person with an ileo-anal pouch, who needs to empty it at fairly frequent intervals throughout the day), he or she has to 'decide to tell or not to, to let on or not too, to lie or not to lie' (Goffman 1963). In support groups, interactions with others who share the stigma allow the sharing of knowledge, mutual acceptance and moral support that was not available from those who had not shared these experiences (Saylor & Yoder 1988).

Social support networks

The image that we hold of our body is formed and developed primarily through our relationship with others. Therefore, when body integrity is threatened or changed, personal response will be affected or modified by the perceptions and restrictions of others. An awareness of this factor can be used to advantage in as much that friends and family can be encouraged to demonstrate a positive attitude with a view to promoting self-esteem and a positive self-concept (Rafferty 1995).

Individuals who enjoy a rich source of contact (both qualities of relationships) are better able to adapt to the threat of mutilating surgery and an altered pattern of elimination thereafter. Families assist the patient to rejoin social activity, to return to work and to make a positive appraisal of their progress in challenging circumstances (Price 1990). Supportive social networks value the individual whether or not he or she has a changed body image. They provide the setting within which those with an altered body image may be integrated into society and remind them of their personal worth and develop ways of talking comfortably about the changed circumstances (Price 1993).

Whilst it is important for the patient to make the decision to undergo pouch surgery, a partner, family member or significant other may also be included in the preoperative information and counselling given, and the postoperative recovery, moving towards rehabilitation.

Recent research has confirmed that adaptation to stressful events (for example, chronic life-threatening illness) may be facilitated by adequately provided social support (Baider et al 1998). In addition to the family, a supportive network of hospital staff was identified as being of great importance in a patient's adaptation to deformity

(Mulgrew & Dropkin 1991). Therefore part of each intervention with the patient should be assessing how the patient is coping with body image changes and facilitating adaptation.

Self-help groups have also been identified as having an important role. O'Sullivan (1992) found that the majority of patients would have liked to have spoken to someone who had undergone this procedure prior to surgery. As one patient said, 'sitting in someone's house with people the same as me was totally liberating. So many people had had similar experiences' (Norwich Pouch Support Group Member 1997).

Body image and the person with familial adenomatous polyposis (FAP)

The most important feature of this disease is that one or more adenomas in the large bowel will develop into cancer unless prophylactic measures are taken. Surgery is the option of choice, and whereas some patients will undergo an ileorectal anastomosis, others will have a pelvic pouch, as either a first choice or a later one.

FAP is caused by a single autosomal dominant gene; thus, if one parent has the gene, each of the children has a 50 per cent chance of also having it (Black 1997). Although some (without any previous knowledge of their family history) may present in a debilitated condition, regular surveillance is undertaken for people on the FAP register. For this group of patients, it is extremely difficult to agree to major surgery when they feel well, and for them a body image change may be difficult to accept because of this reason.

Body image and the person with ulcerative colitis

Some patients require surgery because of acute disease, whereas others have chronic problems and are unable to enjoy good health. Common problems encountered in this condition are bleeding, diarrhoea, mucous discharge, urgency, abdominal discomfort, anorexia and weight loss, and soreness. An increased incidence of colorectal cancer in patients with long-standing ulcerative colitis has long been recognized, and careful surveillance is necessary, often leading to surgery (Oakley 1991). Thus, this group of patients may undergo a multiplicity of body image problems associated with their disease.

Chronic illness is a lived experience (Cameron & Gregor 1987, cited in Price 1996). Other authors (Bleeker & Mulderij 1992) point out that, in illness, the body 'loses its silence', calling attention to itself. Everyday habits of ignoring the body are no longer possible, and individuals are forced to manage the physical functions in a way that would seem fussy and strange to their healthy peers. This may be evident in patients with ulcerative colitis because of, for example, the weight loss, anorexia, abdominal pain and urgent or frequent diarrhoea encountered.

In Beitz's (1999) study of respondents with an ileo-anal reservoir, the 'restricted life world' category included wishes by the respondents to be free of ulcerative colitis. Their social routines, work and culture were all forcibly altered by the symptoms and signs of their condition. Informants felt that they were being 'chained to the toilet'. Even after receiving an ileo-anal reservoir, the initial response of the body to the neo-rectum involved continued restriction until adaptation progressed.

As one patient stated:

> getting better after a long, chronic illness such as ulcerative colitis can be a very scary thing to do. When you're ill, you long to get your life back, but when you do, you suddenly remember just how different normal life is to cope with. Ulcerative colitis is no beauty treatment – it's bad enough being ill without looking like hell ... I'm not a vain person, no more than anyone I know, but it did matter to me that I lost my looks. It seemed like the final insult. Even now, a year and a half after pouch surgery, I still have a hang-up about how I look, because I'm still dealing with the legacy of ulcerative colitis. (Walls 1997)

Similarly, 'Sarah' says that her mum, who had ulcerative colitis for many years, was very self-conscious and would never go anywhere unless she knew that there was a toilet nearby (Norwich Pouch Support Group Member 1997).

Body image and the person with a permanent stoma

The literature relating to the experience of people with a stoma and their subsequent adaptation to perceived body image changes reveals a number of common themes, for example the difficulties experienced in coming to terms with an ostomy (Dyk & Sunderland 1956, Druss et al 1968, Devlin et al 1971, Eardley et al 1976, Carolan 1984, Salter 1992). Individuals with stomas often have poor psychosocial outcomes, which range from failure to return to occupations and withdrawal from social and intimate contact, to depression and anxiety (McDonald & Anderson 1984). The creation of a stoma represents a physical alteration, which may result in ostomists having poor self-concept and reduced self-esteem (Nordstrum 1988). Those with a stoma very often perceive themselves to be less sexually attractive to their partner (Rolstad et al 1985).

Although most patients with a permanent stoma adapt well psychosocially (Rolstad & Nemer 1985) approximately 20 per cent experience long-term difficulty (Dozois et al 1980). It is important to bear in mind that patients coming for pouch surgery do so because they do not want to have a permanent stoma. In the small percentage of patients in whom the pouch 'fails', however, it becomes necessary to fashion a permanent stoma, and patients will need much support in their disappointment and their coming to terms with an ileostomy for life. The next section describes how this experience differs from that of a person with a temporary stoma.

Body image and the person with a temporary ileostomy

Some patients will routinely have a temporary stoma as part of the operative procedure when constructing a pelvic pouch. This is because the pouch may be constructed as a one-, two- or three-stage procedure, stages two and three incorporating a stoma. Controversy exists over whether the temporary stoma can be omitted. Some randomized studies have shown that it can be safely avoided in carefully selected patients (Grobler et al 1992).

Patients need to be aware that because a reservoir is created with about 35 cm or more of small intestine (Strader 1989), other authors suggesting that 58 cm be used (McGonagle 1988), the temporary ileostomy arises from the mid-ileum. For the first few days after surgery, therefore, there may be a high volume of watery output, the effluent generally being more fluid than that seen with an end-ileostomy.

The reservoir population do not, however, represent an average group of patients with stomas because their stoma is temporary. They experience increased morbidity with loop ileostomy and do not have a commitment to the stoma (Rolstad & Nemer 1985). Incorporating the stoma, albeit temporarily, into their body image is important, and nursing care should be sensitive and patient-focused.

If for any reason the patient has to keep the temporary stoma longer than anticipated, he or she may need support in learning to adapt.

Body image and the person with a pelvic pouch

The pelvic pouch operation involves the removal of the whole of the large intestine as well as the rectum. The muscles surrounding the anus are left intact, but the lining of the narrow anal canal is stripped away so that the whole of the disease is removed (Keighley 1990). The great attraction of the pelvic pouch operation is that these patients use the normal route of defecation, and the average patient will empty the pouch about five times in 24 hours, urgency rarely being a complaint (Oresland 1996). Following pouch surgery, the anal sphincter is, however, usually weaker and needs time to recover, which can be a testing time for the patient and family (Maxwell, undated). Some people may need to evacuate the pouch at night, or there may be nocturnal soiling, and this can have an effect on a patient's body image.

The time from the first operation until reservoir adaptation has been estimated to be about 6–12 months. During this period, people can return to school, work and their usual activities (Rolstad & Rothenberger, undated). Results for the operation (bearing in mind that patients may be biased towards feeling that the pouch operation has been worthwhile) have shown that about 90 per cent think that their quality of life is better after pouch surgery, based on aspects such as body image, clothing, sport, work and sexual appeal (Nicholls & Harocopas 1990). With the pouch procedure, long-term body image adaptation will be minimized (Nemer & Rolstad 1985).

In Beitz's (1999) study, over half the respondents reported altered pelvic sensation after pouch surgery. In particular, they could feel the reservoir filling after they had eaten a meal. They also reported more noticeable peristaltic sounds. However, the pouch had a major positive impact on the body image of both male and female respondents, allowing them to feel that they were no longer patients.

Comparison between a stoma and an ileo-anal pouch

The literature addressing the effects of body image changes in patients undergoing conventional stomas compared with continent pouches suggests that, in the main, people with continent procedures feel more satisfied with their body image and sexuality than those with a conventional stoma, also reporting that the ileo-anal reservoir enhanced their lives (Nicholls 1983, Rolstad et al 1985, Pemberton 1988, Everett 1989, Salter 1995/6, Bond et al 1997).

Salter's (1992) qualitative study found that patients with a continent pouch, provided they were not experiencing difficulties with the pouch, were of the opinion that such a procedure was preferable to an ileostomy. In examining these patients soon after pouch surgery, it was, however, found that the majority still considered their experience to be traumatic. This implies that the benefits of a continent pouch were not entirely obvious as body image changes resulting from stoma surgery still had a perceived negative effect on the patients. This affected the outcome of the study so that the differences between the two groups of patient were not as significant as was perceived by the author. In this small study, however, three respondents talked about not feeling 'normal' whilst they had a stoma, comparing this to feelings of normality with a pouch.

In considering quality of life, one study found that all but 1 out of 54 patients were unequivocal in preferring their quality of life after restorative proctocolectomy over that of their previous ileostomy. The advantages of the reservoir most cited in Nicholls' (1983) study included greater confidence, ease of management and the feeling of being more 'normal'. Similarly, Pemberton et al (1987), in an examination of seven areas of daily activities, revealed that a continent procedure was associated with improved performance in each category.

The pouch offers the patient greater potential for the best possible quality of life by obviating the need for a permanent ileostomy, thus enhancing body image (Golligher 1983). Therefore satisfaction with the pouch procedure has been high. The absence of a permanent ileostomy has eliminated many body image problems, and sexual function following this procedure has not been a major problem (Rolstad & Rothenberger, undated, Nemer & Rolstad 1985)

Some authors, state Bond et al (1997), have also reported an acceptable quality of life after a restorative proctocolectomy (Kohler et al 1992, O'Sullivan 1992, Sagar et al 1993) compared with after an ileostomy. In Bond et al's study, 72 per cent of respondents who had received an ileostomy as part of the operative procedure for a pouch were asked whether or not they would have preferred to keep it. The pouch was overwhelmingly seen as being preferable. There was no correlation of gender, age, occupation and anal soreness with perceived quality of life.

Other studies (for example, Kohler & Troidl 1995) have, however, attributed an improvement in quality of life to the colectomy rather than the restorative nature of the operation (Weinryb et al 1995). Indeed, Weinryb et al suggest that the type of surgery, be it ileostomy or pouch, may not affect quality of life, but the eradication of the disease itself is important.

It is believed that there is a 'cost' involved whether patients have a stoma or a pouch. The cost regarding the stoma concerns the inability to control output and the need to wear an appliance. The costs to people undergoing pelvic pouch formation are those of normally requiring more than one operation, complications such as pouchitis that may result from the procedure and the frequency of having their bowels open (Salter 1992a).

Sexuality

The expressions of human sexuality and body image are virtually inseparable within both health and illness (McKenzie 1988), and as human beings we express ourselves sexually throughout our lives from birth to death. Sexuality therefore encompasses much more than the physical act of intercourse, involving instead the totality of being human (Webb 1984).

It is feared that nurses still have difficulty in addressing the sexual needs of patients and that people who present for care do not leave their sexuality at home any more than they leave their fear behind (Wells 1990). Wells further challenges us by suggesting that we mouth platitudes about activities of daily living, but how often do we mention sexuality in care plans?

Patients are not expected to care for a surgical wound or injury, so it is unfair to deny them help and information in adjusting and responding to changes in sexuality (Webb & O'Neill 1989). Although we, as health-care professionals, need to acknowledge our own biases and prejudices, we need not ignore our own beliefs or standards of mortality but should seek to be non-judgemental in our approach (Webb 1984).

So how do health-care professionals incorporate a discussion of sexuality into patient care? Do nurses believe that it is appropriate to discuss sexuality only with patients whose disease or surgery will have a direct impact on their sexual function (in terms of, for example, impotence after rectal surgery), or do they feel that, as health educators, they should invite all patients to discuss any concerns about sexuality that they may have (Salter 1992b)? The majority of nurses in one study did not believe that sexual counselling was a part of care, leaving the question of which other health-care professionals may include this as part of their role. If discussions about sexuality were to become as much a regular part of nursing as wound care or nutrition, nurses' confidence and skill in handling such problems would improve (Webb & O'Neill 1989).

The personal nature of sexuality makes some argue that providing information is an invasion of privacy. It is, however, precisely because patients may find this an issue difficult to discuss that the nurse should indicate that sexuality is a legitimate subject for discussion. 'How are things?' or 'How are things between you and your partner?' are a little vague, but they are non-intrusive and might therefore be successful in eliciting a response. The nurse might instead try something more direct: 'Some patients with a condition like yours have questions or concerns about sex or sexuality. I was wondering whether you had any questions you might like to discuss with me or someone else.' The latter is direct but courteous and opens the door for the nurse and patient to begin a discussion (Gamlin 1999).

Discussion can be facilitated by using patient information booklets, which usually include information on sexual issues (Salter 1992b). Nurses could start discussing issues of sexuality with patients as part of the assessment process.

The assessment of sexual health begins with taking a sexual history, questions (adapted from McPheteridge 1968) include:

• Has having an illness or treatment interfered with your role as a parent or spouse?
• Has your treatment changed the way in which you see yourself as a man or woman?

- Has your treatment caused any changes in sexual functioning?
- Do you expect your sex life to be changed in any way after discharge from hospital?

One of the most important factors in total sexual rehabilitation for patients is an educated and informed partner (Lomont et al 1978). The patient must first, however, identify the partner. Is he or she, for example, in a heterosexual or homosexual relationship, or is the person bisexual? Furthermore, it is widely agreed that the quality of a sexual relationship after a patient's illness is more strongly related to the previous quality of the relationship than to any other factors. It is therefore of great importance to include the partner (with the patient's permission) in patient education and decision-making.

Health-care professionals frequently focus on the patient's sexuality and overlook the effects that the illness may have on the partner. The healthy partner can experience fatigue as a result of the extra roles that he or she may have to adopt during the patient's illness and recovery. It is also common for the healthy partner to feel hesitant about initiating the sexual relationship with the ill person. The healthy partner may be afraid of imposing his or her advances on the person who is unwell, and the ill partner may take this as rejection (Salter 1992b). Communication is thus of paramount importance, the nurse being well placed to facilitate this area of care.

As with encountering body image problems, patients with a history of ulcerative colitis may feel that the disease has had an effect on how they perceive themselves sexually. This may be attributed to the chronicity of inflammatory bowel disease, whereas the patient with FAP may not, on the whole, have had overt problems in this area. The person with a stoma may perceive him or herself to be less sexually attractive (Rolstad & Rothenberger, undated, Nemer & Rolstad 1985, Salter 1992), but some studies have found that the majority have adapted (Burnham et al 1997).

Sexuality and the person with an internal pouch

Whereas, in the creation of a stoma, the physiological alteration may result in patients perceiving themselves to be less sexually attractive and desirable to their partner, studies have shown that a continent procedure improves the quality of sexual life in about 85 per cent of both men and women (Nicholls et al 1983). It is, however, important to ask (especially when it is, in the main, younger patients who undergo surgery for FAP or inflammatory bowel disease) whether patients, irrespective of the type of operation, undergo sexual difficulties (Oresland 1996). In considering the effect of a pouch on personal relationships, particularly sexual relationships, Bond et al (1997) found that the results were, overall, positive, almost three-quarters reporting an improvement in their sex life.

For patients undergoing pelvic pouch surgery, sexual relations may be resumed when the person feels comfortable, that is, when the abdominal incision has healed and the tenderness has subsided (Borwell 1997). Both men and women almost always achieve normal function after pouch surgery. After any major operation in this area, it may, however, take some time before libido returns, and for women there may be discomfort with intercourse in the first couple of months (Maxwell, undated). Similarly, if men have erection or ejaculation difficulties, advice should be given to convalescence before attempting sexual intercourse. When considering homosexual patients, counselling should encourage the person to refrain from anal sex after pelvic pouch construction: anal intercourse can stretch and damage the sphincter muscles, which can lead to incontinence and leakage (Borwell 1997). It is important for the nurse to provide support in this vital aspect of sexuality care and to assess for any difficulties that may be encountered. Referral to an appropriate sexual counsellor should be considered if difficulties persist for the patient and/or partner.

Sexuality concerns, especially in women, have received little attention. Some women feel more sexual, whereas others have decreased desire (Hull & Erwin-Toth 1996). Vaginal discharge and dyspareunia are well-known problems in patients with proctocolectomy and conventional ileostomy but seem less common in pelvic pouch patients. The reason for this lies in the anatomical changes that take place after proctocolectomy, when the vagina and the uterus fall back and adhere to the sacrum. The posterior dislocation is prevented in pelvic pouch patients if the pouch replacing the rectum is interposed between the sacrum and the internal genitals (Oresland 1996).

Altered sexual function caused by pelvic dissection to remove the rectum may, however, occur, and the associated changes, including retrograde ejaculation, impotence, dyspareunia and vaginal dryness, may be lifelong (Fazio et al 1995, Bambrick et al 1996). Preoperative counselling and postoperative support are essential to inform patients about these possible problems and to help them cope with the consequences (Hull 1999). Male patients, in particular, must be permitted to express their anxieties related to impotence preoperatively. Discussions on sexual intimacy should be appropriately timed and occur only after basic physiological needs have been met postoperatively (Beitz 1999).

Many women receiving a pelvic pouch are young and have concerns about becoming pregnant. An issue frequently raised by women pertains to their future abilities to conceive and carry a pregnancy to term (O'Connor et al 1998). Similarly, men may worry about their ability to father a child after pouch surgery, so there are family planning issues for both sexes. As stated earlier, it is important that the patient recovers physically from surgery and from any effects of previous inflammatory bowel disease that may have led to chronic debilitation. It may be that the patient and partner are eager to plan and start a pregnancy, but it is best if they defer this until an optimal state of health has been reached.

Pregnancy following pelvic reservoir is usually possible but, optimally, should be discussed with the surgeon. Once pregnancy has been achieved, the pelvic location of the pouch may raise concerns in patients and physicians regarding the effect of the enlarging uterus on pouch function and the best way to deliver the infant (O'Connor et al 1998). Surgeons may therefore advise a caesarean section. Whereas normal vaginal delivery is possible, a caesarean section avoids the risk to the pelvic floor muscles and nerves, and prevents the possibility of needing an episiotomy during delivery (Borwell 1997). Successful delivery after ileo-pouch construction has occurred by both vaginal and caesarean section (Hoyman & Rolstad 1992).

O'Connor et al's (1998) study to evaluate pregnancy, delivery and functional results for women who have undergone a pouch procedure showed that 12 women out of 330 who had undergone the pouch procedure between 1982 and 1994 were identified as having at least one pregnancy and delivery. The study concluded that pregnancy and delivery do not affect long-term pelvic pouch function in most patients. The obstetric outcome in most women with a pelvic pouch is good. This study also found that there are no data to support one particular route of delivery over the other. It is important to bear in mind that evidence also suggests that some patients' fertility may be considerably reduced after surgery for inflammatory bowel disease (Oresland 1996).

The nurse's role

The nurse is in a strategic position to address the body image and sexuality needs of patients both before and after surgery. The role of the nurse, in particular the stoma care/pouch nurse, concerns active involvement in comprehensive education. Supportive counselling is fundamental to minimizing complications and facilitating adaptation (Rolstad & Nemer 1985). Patients are willing to undergo multiple surgery to avoid a permanent stoma and will need adequate time for help (Borwell 1997). Whether the patient has decided to have surgery or is at the information-gathering stage, the primary function of the nurse is to provide the information necessary to make informed decisions and to reduce the fear and anxiety aroused by the prospect of surgery (Rolstad & Nemer 1985).

Beitz (1999) suggests that patients distance themselves from bodies that they cannot control and that render them socially unacceptable. She proposes that nurses also need to permit patients with an internal pouch to distance themselves from their bodies psychologically until they are ready to adjust to the new situation.

Preoperative care for pouch surgery

Pre- and postoperative counselling aims to return the patient to the lifestyle enjoyed prior to surgery or, for patients with inflammatory bowel disease, to the situation before their life was limited by the chronicity of such a disease. Pre- and post-operative care sets out to enable the patient to cope both psychologically and physically with the surgery.

The ideal candidates for the pelvic pouch procedure are motivated, relatively healthy patients, with mucosal ulcerative colitis or FAP. Patients should be relatively slender and should have good, competent sphincters (Hull & Erwin-Toth 1996). Patients with FAP normally feel quite well, and surgery may come as a shock to them. Patients with a flare-up of ulcerative colitis will undergo minimal investigations to prevent further damage to the colon. Any preoperative intervention may, however, be embarrasing and humiliating. Patients, whatever their diagnosis or health status, may feel undignified when undergoing rectal examinations. Similarly, the pouchogram (an X-ray of the pouch to check for healing) is undertaken via a small tube. This is rapid and painless but nevertheless undignified (Maxwell, undated factsheet). Body image concerns, such as ensuring that patients are covered with a sheet or blanket as much as possible during procedures, need to be addressed.

For patients undergoing surgery, the preparation and general anaesthetic will represent a loss of control over body activities. Physical changes after surgery can vary from a small scar to mutilation that is sometimes seen as unbearable (Blackmore 1988). For many patients, having surgery is a further assault to their body image. Some things, for example being hospitalized, being shaved and getting into an operating gown, are minor and standard procedures to the health-care professional, but to many of our patients they represent a fear of the unknown, and the fragility of their body image may make them feel even more vulnerable.

Postoperative considerations following ileo-anal pouch surgery

The postoperative period may be particularly difficult in that patients may be exhausted by the number of times that they may need to empty the pouch, with resulting perianal soreness; the role of the nurse in supporting the patient through this period is particularly important. Washing and drying the skin thoroughly and using a barrier cream helps to minimize this problem. The sensation of wanting to defaecate is often relieved by sitting on the lavatory at regular internals to expel mucous from the pouch (Nicholls & Harocopas 1990). The patient may wonder if all this is worth it and will need support at this time.

Core care plans or integrated care pathways can be utilized in individual patient care to allow a holistic approach. In care-planning, nursing intervention can be that of encouraging the patient to express their feelings towards changes to physical appearance and body function. It may help to enhance other areas of the body, with, for example, make-up or particular clothes, which can detract from the altered body image (Batchelor et al 1991). Professional nurses strive to deliver individualized, comprehensive care to their patients, the aim of nursing intervention being to maximize the health potential of patients in our care (Erwin-Toth & Spencer 1991). Those nurses who truly understand their patients may be able to help them to make some sense of and adjust to their new self.

Nurses should offer care that is participative, collaborative and empowering, that is a partnership rather than subordination, one that incorporates reflection and evaluation (Corner 1998). Empowering is about nurses working with patients to understand, assess and teach clients about the altered physiology of their body whilst understanding the experience of this, as described by the patient and family (Price 1996). We should be patient focused, looking at care as a problem or need rather than a symptom or treatment. Therapeutic nursing should be orientated towards illness and its meaning, encouraging illness narratives from the patient and a relationship that is creative rather than passive. This may mean restructuring services to permit such an approach, something that may well need careful investigation in light of current staff shortages and a lack of other resources (Corner 1998).

Nurse education needs to ensure that the nurse acquires competencies in these vital aspects of care. Part of the rehabilitation process includes encouraging patients to view themselves as 'normal' after surgery. Rehabilitation should include the patient, partner and significant others, and should be an enabling process on the part of the nurse.

The crucial role of the nurse in assisting the patient to cope exerts an important impact on quality of survival. It is the perceived nursing activities that affirm patient self-worth and help psychological well-being, body image and social concerns (Padill & Grant 1985). Nurses can make a measurable difference in facilitating adaptations to body images changes. One of the end-products of the nurse's role in the care of the patients with a pouch is to instil into them the belief that they are loved for who they are rather than what they look like or how they feel as a result of their changed physiological function. By working with patents to enable them to live life as they choose. As nurses, we have the privilege of making the difference to patient care and focusing on the patient.

Conclusion

In conclusion, therefore, it is important to state that the pouch is not presented as a 'cure-all' and that patients can make an informed choice about the type of treatment for which they opt (Bond et al 1997). Only one-third of patients escape significant complications, between 5 and 10 per cent of pouches failing and requiring conversion to an end-stoma (Cohen et al 1985, Oresland et al 1996, Becker et al 1991, Fazio et al 1995). Yet despite these obvious drawbacks, patients are still keen to undergo restorative proctocolectomy (Bond et al 1997), the majority of patients electing to have an ileo-anal reservoir again (Rolstad & Nemer 1985). Whether a pouch is sustained for life depends on a number of factors, including sphincter control and complications such as pouchitis, but it is appropriate for the patients themselves to have the last word.

'However, living with a pouch internal or external is a remarkable alternative to the way we were' (Hyams 1996). Another patient (Norwich Pouch Support Group Member 1997) wrote about her 'journey', saying that 'it was not voluntary ... I didn't know it was going to be a major and most significant part of my life. Nor did I know that along the way I would suffer enormous loss and great pain, but that eventually I would meet new people, go on to develop stronger relationships and gain greater knowledge of myself'.

As one member of the Red Lion Group in Norwich (Norwich Pouch Support Group Member 1997) stated, 'It is my view that patients need help to heal from within, not just their bodies but their hearts and minds too ... I may not be the best example of a Park's pouch patient, but most importantly I have come to terms with who I am and what I have to give to others.'

CHAPTER 11

Children and internal pouches

GAIL FITZPATRICK, PAT COLDICUTT AND JULIA WILLIAMS

Children and adolescents with inflammatory bowel disease and familial adenomatous polyposis (FAP) present unique challenges to all health-care professionals involved in their care. From the literature, it is evident that both ulcerative colitis and FAP are being recognized earlier and more frequently (Telander et al 1981, Ziv et al 1995). Restorative proctocolectomy remains the surgical option of choice for this group of patients, and it is important for the nurse to have an understanding of the plight of the young child or adolescent who is contemplating internal pouch surgery.

Ulcerative colitis in children

Ulcerative colitis is one of the two common chronic inflammatory bowel diseases that affect the colon of children. The disease can occur at any time during infancy and childhood, and is far more common than Crohn's disease in children less than 6 years old (Ament et al 1988). The Jewish population outside Israel is at far greater risk of developing the condition than any other ethnic group, although the reason for this is unknown. The chance of a family member developing the condition is 2–3 times greater than that of the general population. The disease is classified as moderate to severe in two-thirds of children as opposed to less than one-third of adults.

It is not difficult to recognize inflammatory bowel disease, even in children, when it presents with classical symptoms such as bloody diarrhoea, abdominal pain and depression (Buller 1997). Not infrequently, these children are diagnosed as being depressed and are seen and treated by psychologists and psychiatrists for different periods of time. In addition to this, several will initially be diagnosed as having a bacterial gastroenteritis with a proven positive faecal culture. It would seem in these cases that colonoscopy is only performed once therapy has failed. Beattie et al (1995, cited in Buller 1997) showed that, in children seen for chronic abdominal pain, a simple routine blood test including a full blood count and erythrocyte sedimentation rate are almost always abnormal in children with inflammatory bowel disease.

Diagnostic testing must include three stool cultures negative for bacterial and viral pathogens, as well as other intestinal parasites, and the absence of *Clostridium difficile* and its toxin in the stool. Flexible sigmoidoscopy and/or colonoscopy should be carried out in every case with biopsies. A barium enema is contraindicated in the severely ill patient because of the risk of perforation of the bowel.

Ulcerative colitis is usually diagnosed in young adults, approximately 2 per cent occurring in children aged 0–9 years and 14 per cent in those between the ages of 10 and 19 (Jackson & Grand 1991). Adolescence is an important stage of growth and development for any child. Adolescent growth proceeds at an amazing rate, the most rapid of any postnatal time (the average weight increment during the adolescent growth spurt being 16 g a day for females and 19 g a day for males; Maloney 1995). It is also during this phase that the skeletal mineral accretion is completed, the peak bone mass being vital for skeletal maintenance and the prevention of osteoporosis.

In addition to the general symptom presentation of ulcerative colitis, the adolescent with chronic disease will also present with anorexia, weight loss and growth retardation. Decreased growth velocity is the most important problem, approximately 14 per cent of patients showing a decreased height per centile at the time of diagnosis. These adolescents also demonstrate delayed sexual maturation with lower measured urinary gonadotropin levels.

Growth retardation is probably related to the intestinal inflammation, malabsorption, anorexia and diarrhoea, with resulting poor nutrition. Nutrient requirements are also increased by the metabolic demands of inflammation, fever and excessive diarrhoea. These nutrient requirements need to be added to those already imposed by adolescent growth. Any deficits in energy or protein may appear insignificant, yet a deficit of as little as 100 kcal a day becomes clinically apparent when the deficit continues daily over several months (Jackson & Grand 1991). Insufficient nutrient intake also inhibits gonadotropin and gonadal steroid secretion, stopping or delaying the onset of pubertal development.

Following diagnosis, medical therapy is initiated, aiming to suppress active inflammation and then maintain remission in order to try to preserve the child's colon. Because of the limited number of clinical trials of therapy in children, most of the treatment guidelines and practices are derived from adult studies.

The mainstay drugs available for treatment are corticosteroids, sulphasalazine, azathioprine, 6-mercaptopurine, methotrexate, ciclosporin, metronidazole and ciprofloxacin. The doses and combinations of drugs used in treatment are determined by the severity of the disease. Consequently, the larger the drug doses and number of drugs used, the greater the potential for drug side-effects. Unfortunately, 50 per cent of adolescent patients have pancolitis at presentation, as opposed to 25–30 per cent of adults (Murrary & Leichtner 1997). Therefore, 50 per cent of adolescents with ulcerative colitis are commenced on high doses of corticosteroids and accompanying drugs.

The most problematic side-effects in relation to adolescent growth and development derive from high-dose or prolonged steroid therapy, which has the potential to cause adrenal suppression, hypertension, fluid retention, acne, hirsutism, cutaneous striae, moon facies, masking of infection, depression, central obesity and growth impairment (Murrary & Leichtner 1997). Growth impairment may occur in the presence or absence of steroid therapy: although there is evidence that corticosteroids may suppress growth velocity, their use in controlling the disease often permits growth to resume at normal rate.

It has been well documented that children have the ability to accelerate their growth when recovering from a growth-impaired period, that is, chronic disease, a phenomenon termed 'catch-up' (Jackson & Grand 1991). Whether or not the catch-up growth during high-dose steroid treatment is sufficient to reach the premorbid growth percentile is unclear. In some patients, disease activity may be controlled by alternate-day low-dose steroid treatment without significant adverse effects on growth. Over time, patients with long-term disease may never catch up and may always have a height stunted below the relevant percentiles, yet they may have the correct weight for their height (Figure 11.1).

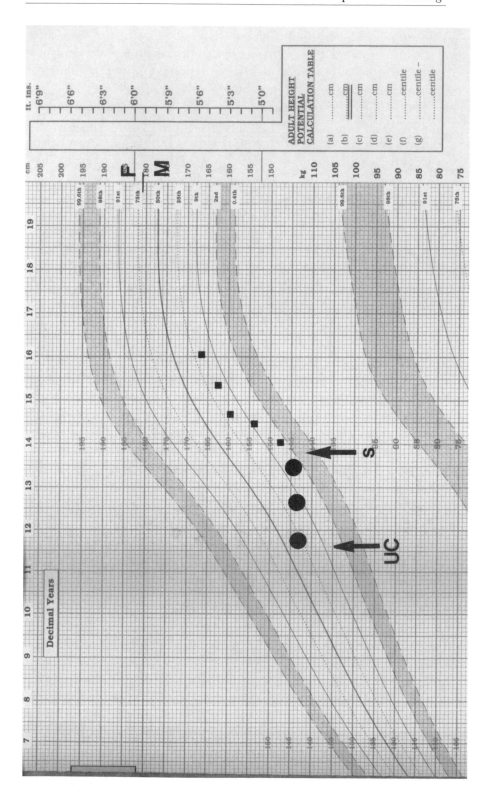

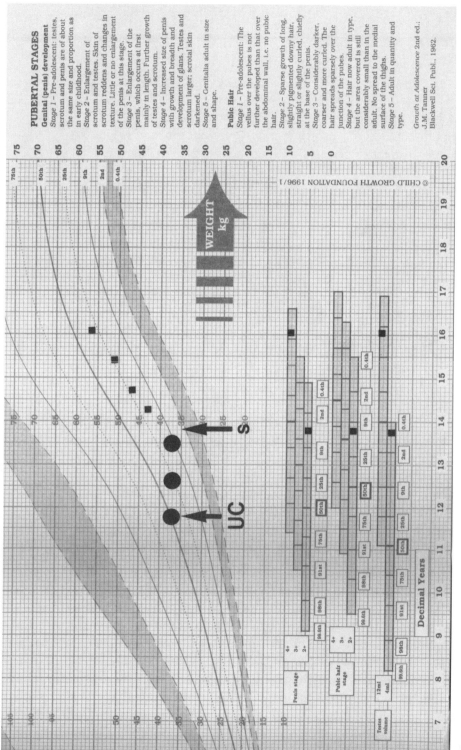

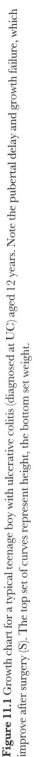

Figure 11.1 Growth chart for a typical teenage boy with ulcerative colitis (diagnosed at UC) aged 12 years. Note the pubertal delay and growth failure, which improve after surgery (S). The top set of curves represent height, the bottom set weight.

The steroid treatment tends to produce emotional changes, with feelings of inferiority and depression in adolescent patients, not helped by having the additional problem of coping with changes in their body image caused by steroid treatment, that is, striae, facial mooning, central obesity, acne and hirsutism. The adolescent period is already a traumatic time for any youngster.

Adolescents are constantly comparing themselves with their peers and feel threatened if they are in any way different, often isolating themselves from their friends. During this period, adolescents with ulcerative colitis also become aware of their peers entering puberty, watching them develop and change in appearance. This only highlights even more that they are different as their sexual maturation is somewhat slower, resulting in increased feelings of isolation and depression.

Adolescents with ulcerative colitis usually tolerate their disease, drug therapy and hospital admissions but over a period of time find their altered appearance as a result of the steroid therapy difficult to cope with. Any adolescent requiring prolonged drug therapy should be considered for surgical treatment, including the option of an internal pouch. During these discussions, the adolescent's psychological state and personal views should always be taken into account.

Buller (1997) highlights the potential benefits of nutritional therapy and recommends serious consideration for nutritional therapy in addition to aggressive medical therapy. Some studies have shown the benefit of nocturnal nasogastric feeding via an infusion pump to supplement the daily intake. Importantly, nutritional support has been shown to be as effective as steroids in achieving disease remission in children. Furthermore, no significant differences have been shown in studies using elemental diets versus polymeric diets (Buller 1997).

It is widely acknowledged that, in chronic cases of ulcerative colitis, surgery leads to improved linear growth and prolonged symptom-free periods in most children and adolescents (Nicholls et al 1995).

FAP is a rare disorder, accounting for fewer than 1 per cent of colorectal carcinomas in adults (Phillips et al 1993). Since FAP is a potentially preventable cause of colorectal carcinoma, clinicians should have an adequate knowledge of it in order to identify the disease and manage the patient and family (see Chapter 2).

FAP is an autosomal dominant, inherited disorder characterized by the development of many hundreds or thousands of adenomatous polyps in the colon and rectum, which can undergo malignant change. The children of an affected individual carry a 50 per cent risk of inheriting the predisposing gene. Hoffenberg et al (1999) suggest that the clinical spectrum of symptomatic polyps and the frequency of FAP are not well defined in children, concluding that juvenile polyposis coli is common in children with symptomatic polyps and is associated with anaemia, right-colon polyps and adenomas. They suggest that the risk of polyps and colorectal cancer in the relatives of those with juvenile polyposis coli requires further study.

For a child who is aware that his or her parent is a known gene carrier, screening is likely to occur from the early teens. This is when it is felt that the onset of the disease occurs, symptoms of the disease presenting between the ages of 25 and 30 and the median age for the development of colonic cancer being 35–40 years. The age at which colonic surveillance begins reflects the natural history of the disease. An onset of polyp formation and cancer in childhood is very unusual, but there has been a recent association with a specific genetic mutation (Eccles 1997). When a childhood onset of polyps (Figure 11.2) has occurred, other children at risk in the family must be offered earlier genetic testing and endoscopic surveillance.

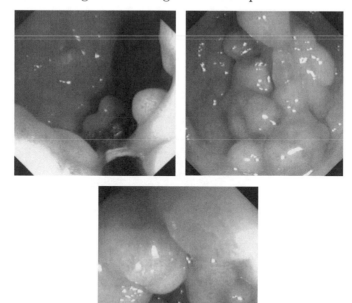

Figure 11.2 Juvenile polyps. Many polyps can be seen in the upper, mid and lower rectum, requiring this 14-year-old girl to undergo a colectomy and pouch procedure (see Plate 14).

Table 11.1 Experiences of ileo-anal pouches in children

	Telander et al (1990) (n = 121)	Fonkalsrud et al (1992) (n = 82)	Davis et al (1994) (n = 30)	Eckhoff et al (1994) (n = 19)	Romanos et al (1996) (n = 15)
Diagnosis					
UC	101	67	28	9	12
FAP	19	14	2	10	2
Other	1	1	0	0	1
Median age in years (range)	15 (3–29)	14.6 (6–18)	14 (5–16)	15.3 (11–18)	15 (6–17)
Procedure					
Straight restorative proctocolectomy	49	6	–	–	2
'J' pouch	72	–	16	–	7
'S' pouch	–	–	14	–	4
'W' pouch	–	–	–	19	1
Lateral ileal reservoir	–	76	–	–	
Morbidity					
Pelvic sepsis	4	–	1	–	
Small bowel obstruction	20	10	3	3	3
Ileo-anal stenosis	7	14	1	2	1
Fistulas	14	3	–	–	
Pouch stasis	–	30	–	–	
Other	9	0	2	–	5
Pouch failure	6	7	0	0	0
Pouch revision	0	19	0	0	2
Pouchitis (%)	22	–	27	21	42
Function					
Stool frequency (per 24 hours)	5	3–5	4	3	4
Continence (approx. %)					
Normal	55	85	70	90	80
Minor	40	15	30	10	20
Moderate	5	–	–	–	–

Surgical options

The surgical option of choice is undoubtedly restorative proctocolectomy, other surgical options that may be considered in selected patients including proctocolectomy with either a Brooke ileostomy or a Kock pouch, colectomy with ileorectal anastomosis, and mucosal proctectomy and ileo-anal pull-through (Romanos et al 1996). Surgery, when indicated, is curative if a proctocolectomy is carried out; however, the timing and choice of the surgical procedure require both experience and expert surgical judgement.

Children undergo colorectal surgery because of urgent problems, either because they have chronic disease that has failed medical management or because of the risk of malignancy (Telander et al 1981). The choice of operation requires a consideration of the advantages and disadvantages of a particular procedure and must be tailored to the individual child's or adolescent's needs and circumstances (Frizelle & Burt 1997). The complications of pouch surgery are generally the same as are seen in adults (Table 11.1). Most children are determined to maintain the function of their pouch; if complications persist, especially in the pre-pubertal period, it may be appropriate to defunction the pouch until such time as they become young adults, when they can make their own decisions for their future.

The choice between restorative proctocolectomy and ileorectal anastomosis in the treatment of ulcerative colitis and FAP remains controversial (Karthenser et al 1996). Ileorectal anastomosis effectively leaves the 'diseased' rectum in situ, and fashioning an ileorectal anastomosis requires a quiescent or minimally inflamed rectum if the procedure is to be successful. The functional results vary and greatly depend on rectal compliance and the extent and activity of the original disease. Regular surveillance of the rectum is necessary as the risk of recurrent disease, including malignancy, is increased. Where recurrence occurs, secondary proctectomy and pouch formation can be safely offered to patients with an ileorectal anastomosis and a high risk of rectal carcinoma (Penna et al 1993). Ileorectal anastomosis is, however, recommended in the surgical treatment of chronic ulcerative colitis in children (Orkin et al 1990).

Mucosal proctectomy and ileo-anal pull-through is increasingly used in children requiring total colectomy for ulcerative colitis or

FAP (Shamberger et al 1994). This procedure has also been the surgical management of total colonic Hirschsprung's disease in infants and children (Coran 1990). Functional results are reported as 4–8 bowel movements per day, with a median of four (Shamberger et al 1994). Minimal nocturnal incontinence is reported (Shamberger et al 1999), the main complications being ileo-anal stenosis, an elongated ileal spout, outflow obstruction and intestinal obstruction (Fonkalsrud & Loar 1992). Overall, the ileo-anal pull-through is seen as an excellent surgical option for children with ulcerative colitis and FAP, producing minimal, if any, adverse effects on their long-term quality of life (Shamberger et al 1999).

Considerations during and after surgery

Special care needs of adolescents in hospital

The vast majority of children who undergo internal pouch surgery fall within the adolescent age group. Adolescents, like all patients, need care tailored to meet their specific needs in order to minimize the possible stresses caused by hospital admission. In 1990, the National Association for the Welfare of Children in Hospital published *Setting Standards for Adolescents in Hospital* (NAWCH 1990) in an attempt to make the hospital environment more suitable for this group (Farrelly 1994). The document states, for example, that adolescents in hospital have a need:

- for psychological as well as medical care;
- to be nursed with others of their age group in a designated area;
- to be treated as individuals;
- to receive support from their family and peer groups;
- to have free access to appropriate recreational activities, such as television, audio equipment and table tennis;
- for privacy – this relates to bathroom facilities as well as to a private place to talk or just be alone;
- for education.

Specialist adolescent units are best equipped to meet adolescents' needs, but in the UK this type of facility remains the exception rather than the rule, and adolescents continue to be nursed on adult or children's wards. As long as this is the case, it is important that nurses caring for them can provide informed and sensitive care catering to their particular needs so that hospital admission can be as untraumatic as possible (Shelley 1993).

Informed consent

Obtaining consent for medical treatment is somewhat more complex in children than in adults. The Family Law Reform Act 1969 stated that, at 16 years of age, a child's consent is as effective as if he or she were an adult. The Children Act 1989 then stated that a child under the age of 16 could refuse to submit to a medical assessment or treatment if 'of sufficient understanding to make an informed decision', in other words if competent to make a valid decision. It is not an easy task to decide whether a child is 'competent', a procedure also known as the 'Gillick test' (Montgomery 1997).

The British Medical Association and the Law Society have produced guidance on assessing competence and suggest that regard should be made to the young patient's ability to understand that there is a choice and that choices have consequences, his or her willingness and ability to make a choice, and the patient's understanding of the nature and purpose of the proposed procedure and the available alternatives, including risks and side-effects (Hendrick 1997).

If the child is felt to be incompetent to make an informed decision, the decision will rest with the parents. If the child is declared 'competent' yet refuses treatment, or the parents refuse to consent to treatment, the medical staff may request authorization from the courts to proceed with treatment. This is given if the child's or parent's decision can be proved to be dangerously unwise and puts the child at risk. Ideally, before proceeding with any treatment, consent should be obtained from the parents and the child.

Bowel preparation

Bowel preparation in children varies from consultant to consultant and hospital to hospital. The preparation for surgery may start prior to admission, using the following regimen. Sodium picosulphate is usually given twice a day 2 days prior to admission. The child is then admitted on the day before surgery and receives clear fluids only. This regimen is considered to be successful when the child is passing clear fluid. Children prior to colonoscopy often require a phosphate enema (the amount depending on age and weight), these not usually being administered to children under 3 years of age.

Bowel preparation tends to be less vigorous nowadays because of the trauma to the child (and parent) and because of the potential electrolyte imbalance post-administration.

Stoma-siting

The aim of siting a stoma is to enable the patient and carer to manage the application of the appliance effectively in order to prevent leakage and allow normal activity to continue. The child's individual needs and activities should be assessed, the siting not being carried out in isolation but in conjunction with preoperative counselling in a language that both child and carer can understand. The area selected should be as flat as possible, avoiding any scars, the umbilicus, the hip bone, the rib cage and the waist line, and should be positioned in a place that is visible to the patient. The stoma care nurse can assess this by placing tape in different positions and asking the patient if he or she can see it; care must obviously be taken in the younger child.

Stoma-siting must be carried out with the child's or parent's consent and in the presence of the parent or guardian. It is normal practice to ensure that the child and parent agree to the final siting before the mark is made. It is also important to document in the child's care plan where the site has been marked, this being signed and dated. Preoperative siting is an important part of stomal surgery and is crucial to the aftercare of patients; it is a skill, and the stoma care nurse is accountable to his or her patients.

Body image and self-esteem

Smith (1984) states that we all have a body image of ourselves that is formed at birth and develops as we grow. Our image is influenced by many factors, such as environment, social and attitudes. Childhood places an enormous significance on peer group approval, wanting to fit in and not being different from the group. Specifically, the adolescent with a temporary loop ileostomy may show distress affecting body image, socialization, peer identity, and emotional and economic independence (Manworren 1996).

Brydolf (1996) identified that adolescents are confronted with problems such as social changes within family and peer groups, and biological and psychological body changes. Thus, living with a condition that could potentially result in stoma formation can have major implications for their physical and emotional development. During adolescence, one's body image is already constantly changed, and this can be an especially difficult time for a child to undergo stoma surgery. For children with ulcerative colitis, there are two schools of thought. One is to form a stoma early on and prevent the change in body image caused by a delay in puberty or poor health. Alternatively, the surgeon can delay creating a stoma during adolescence, but this may in turn result in growth failure if conservative treatment fails, leading to later surgery with stoma formation.

Postoperatively these adolescents thrive, gain weight, grow and may declare that they wish they had had a stoma before. This is not so with everyone, and some may not welcome stoma surgery, even if it means an end to their diarrhoea and pain.

Adolescents are extremely vulnerable both before and after surgery, and if they have a negative body image, their self-esteem will also be low and their coping mechanisms will be affected. Wallace (1993) found that one of the biggest fears of adolescents is that people will avoid them, resulting in loneliness and isolation. The revulsion for the stoma felt by others often decreases their self-esteem, even if it is only perceived rather than actual revulsion. The more significant the person showing the distaste, the more traumatic the situation becomes, so parents and best friends are particularly important in helping to maintain a positive body image.

During hospital appointments and hospital admissions, it is important that both nursing and medical staff consistently portray a realistic yet positive attitude to the stoma surgery and the ultimate internal pouch surgery, with the eventual closure of the stoma. Adolescents wish to know exactly what is going to happen to them, especially in terms of physical outcomes such as scarring and whether they can go to school, play sport, go swimming and wear all the latest fashions.

Time factors are also important when treatment plans are being discussed: adolescents want to know how long they will have to keep the stoma. They will then latch on to the shortest timescale mentioned, and if after that time has elapsed they do not have a date for their stoma to be closed, their acceptance of the stoma tends to reduce and their self-esteem drops. Adolescents are not normally very patient in terms of having to wait for anything, so it is advantageous to over-estimate rather than under-estimate timescales.

To help adolescents to develop a positive body image and high self-esteem, it is a good idea to encourage their friends to visit while they are in hospital as this helps to reduce their feeling of isolation. They often benefit by meeting another person their age who has the same condition. It has been found that the more independent adolescents are in caring for their stoma, the easier it is to return to school and rejoin their peer group, as they feel in control of their situation. Throughout the adolescent's illness, the nursing staff should offer them ample opportunity to express their feelings; in response, they should receive support, encouragement and honest, realistic answers to any questions raised.

Adolescents have a greater risk of depression, although this can happen at any age. Stoddard et al (1992) found that it often occurred once the child had recovered from the illness, that is, following pouch surgery and the closure of the stoma. This delay may be caused by the growing realization of the permanence of operation scars. Girls with abdominal scars have a lower self-esteem and negative body image of themselves than boys. This may be because the media and society place a huge emphasis on physical appearance for girls, whereas boys may pass off scarring as a 'war wound'. It is important never to minimize the effect that scars have on a person's self-esteem; offering waterproof camouflage make-up to cover their scars will have a profound effect on their self-esteem and will give them a positive body image.

Overall, when questioned, most adolescents are 'keen to get on with their lives', doing 'teenage things', and the pouch procedure appears to give them the confidence to do this (Rintala et al 1997).

Pain control

The multidisciplinary team should adopt a child-centred philosophy so that effective pain relief can occur. Nurses should act as the child's advocate, ensuring that the analgesia prescribed is appropriate and effective, and that the child is not subjected to unnecessary pain, such as repeated sessions of blood-taking when 'grouping bloods' means that the child only needs one venepuncture. The use of local anaesthetic cream applied to the skin will also help to allay children's fears prior to venepuncture or cannulation. Preparation in the form of preoperative and pre-procedure teaching and discussions can help to allay children's fears and help them to manage their pain and feel more in control. The play therapist has an important role here.

Epidurals using bupivicaine infusions have been successful in managing postoperative pain in children (Desparmet et al 1990), patient-controlled analgesia being a successful alternative. In this system, the child can operate a pump by a hand-held trigger that, provided the lock-out period has elapsed, signals the pump to deliver a pre-set amount of the drug via the child's infusion line, giving the child control over their analgesia.

Stoma care

When teaching a child how to care for a temporary ileostomy, it is important that the child's parents are, whenever possible, involved. It is, however, important that the teaching is directed at the child, the parent being there as a bystander to offer support and encouragement as needed. Parental attitudes influence the child, some parents tending to promote dependency because they fear the child cannot manage alone and must be protected. The nurse should encourage parents to support the child's efforts to learn the skills of stoma care and become independent. It is well documented that a child who views stoma care as a normal part of daily toilet is more adept at integrating the stoma into his or her self-image.

The child may also require assistance in obtaining support for stoma care at school, so it may be necessary for the stoma care nurse to visit the school in order to educate fellow classmates and teachers, explaining the need for the child to go to the bathroom as required and the child's need for privacy when emptying or changing the appliance. Research has shown that stoma formation between the ages of 6 and 12 years has long-term effects on psychosocial development (Erwin-Toth 1999). Efforts by families, teachers and nurses to promote normalization can ease the initial adjustment, and peer support from other young people with stomas and ileao-anal pouches may help.

Electrolyte depletion

Adolescents with stomas are at risk of sodium depletion from increased gastrointestinal loss; a depletion of this electrolyte may lead to poor weight gain, malaise and even growth failure. It is common practice to measure urinary sodium in these patients and replace losses with either oral rehydration solution or sodium tablets.

Closure of the stoma

The optimal time to close the stoma in children will depend greatly on the age of the child at the time of pouch surgery. If the child is pre-pubertal, thought should be given to closing the stoma once puberty has occurred. The rationale for this is that if sepsis occurs post-closure in the pre-pubertal phase, it is likely to inhibit pubertal growth. It is important that this issue is discussed with the paediatrician, colorectal surgeon and nurse specialist as well as the child and parents in order to plan for the optimal point to close the stoma.

Pouch function

Functional outcome is a major determinant of patient satisfaction with the pouch procedure, and it would appear that pouch function is as good in children as it is in adults (Romanos et al 1996). Several studies have reviewed the experience of ileo-anal pouches in children (see Table 11.1 above) in order to evaluate the outcome and discuss the problems and challenges associated with the procedure.

A pouch frequency of four motions in 24 hours is noted within each study. It would also appear that the morbidity is similar to that of adults. All the studies (Telander et al 1990, Fonkalsrud & Loar 1992, Davis et al 1994, Eckhoff et al 1994, Romanos et al 1996) conclude excellent results with very good function and no stoma. Highlighting their experiences of children who have undergone the pouch procedure ultimately provides important evidence that restorative proctocolectomy is a surgical option worth considering in those children and adolescents with ulcerative colitis or FAP (Durno et al 1998). Romanos et al (1996) express an interest in studying the population of patients with pouches from childhood to determine the survival and functional outcome of the ileao-anal pouch after 30–-40 years.

Effects of hospitalization on family and social life

Having a child in hospital can be extremely traumatic for the child's parents and family. Whenever possible, one parent should stay with the hospitalized child. During the hospital admission, maintaining contact with the rest of the family is vital. Parents often try to arrange to spend some time at home in order to be with their other children. Siblings at home may sometimes become jealous of the sister or brother in hospital, who appears to be getting all the attention. If possible, the whole family should visit together, or the hospitalized child should to be allowed out for a short period so that the family can spend some time together. During and after children's admissions to hospital, it is important for them to maintain contact with their friends. Whilst in hospital, contact can be achieved by encouraging friends to visit, write or telephone. Once home, children should be encouraged to resume their social activities as soon as they are fit to do so.

Education

The chances are that any child with ulcerative colitis will miss a considerable amount of schooling, whether sick at home or admitted to hospital. The fact that a child is ill does not relieve the local education authorities of the duty to comply with statutory requirements to provide education. Every effort should be made to ensure that the interruption to the child's schooling is kept to a minimum (Department of Health 1991). The educational needs of sick children can be met by providing either home or hospital tuition. The aim being to liaise closely with the child's school to ensure continuity and a stable standard of education. If the child is due to take exams or assessments, arrangements can be made for these to take place in the hospital as long as the child is well enough. Maintaining education during long hospital admissions helps to reduce children's fears that they will never be able to catch up on all the work they have missed on return to their school and makes integration back in to school easier.

Once the child is well enough to return to school, careful planning needs to take place so that it can be as smooth as possible. The types of issue that need addressing relate to any additional lessons required for the child to catch up on work missed and arrangements for a private toilet and/or changing area to be available for the child to care for the ileostomy or cope with their frequent toilet needs once the ileostomy has been closed. For younger or less independent children, arrangements needs to be made for a 'carer' to be available at school to provide help and support for their toilet needs. It might also be possible to time the surgery during the school holidays or in a gap year. Each school has a Special Educational Needs Co-ordinator, who will be the one responsible for co-ordinating the arrangements for the child to be integrated back into school once well enough.

Occasionally, integration back in to school does not prove to be so easy, and parents can become confused and baffled by some of the education authorities' red tape. There is a national support group called Network 81, a network of parents who have children with special educational needs, that can help to demystify the situation for these parents (see Useful Addresses).

Financial considerations

The cost of having a child with a chronic illness requiring repeat admission to hospital must never be underestimated. The child is often referred to a regional centre with the expertise to treat the child. Thus, the child and family have to travel long distances for treatment. The overall costs involved are travelling expenses, which need to include the whole family so that they can visit the child in hospital, meals for the parent who wishes to stay with the child, childcare arrangements for siblings left at home or if one or both parents need to have time off work, and so on.

There are various avenues by which to obtain financial support, for example the following:

- The Disability Living Allowance is a tax-free social security benefit for people with an illness or a disability. Application forms can be obtained from any social security office.
- The Family Fund Trust (Caven 1996; see Useful Addresses) was set up by the government in 1973, becoming in 1996 an independent

trust for families with chronically sick children under the age of 16 years. The trust provides grants for certain items related to the child's care needs and also aims to pass on information to families about other available services and benefits. The fund is means-tested, so the family's income and savings must be within the trust's financial guidelines for them to qualify.

If the family are receiving income support, they may be entitled to travel expenses to the hospital for the child and one accompanying adult. There are also local support groups that might also be able to help the family.

Summary

The success rate of the ileo-anal pouch procedure is comparable to that of adults (see Table 11.1 above). It would appear from the literature that the pouch procedure is the choice of operation for children and adolescents who want ileo-anal continuity restored after colectomy for ulcerative colitis or FAP (Durno et al 1998, Romanos et al 1996). It is important that nurses have both the skills and the expertise in paediatric surgical nursing to aid this client group in the decision-making process that will ultimately affect the rest of the lives.

CHAPTER 12

Patients' perspectives

Julia Williams

As editor, I am extremely grateful to the following patients for putting their experiences down on paper. Their stories have not been edited in order to maintain authenticity, but, it is important to note that the text that follows relates to their individual experiences, and information provided is purely anecdotal.

Yvonne's story – Living with an ileo-anal pouch

Even when I developed ulcerative colitis in 1991, a few months before my thirtieth birthday, I never dreamed that the years that followed would be filled with so much pain, grief and uncertainty, but also a period of learning about others and myself.

Up until that time I was a happy-go-lucky young lady who enjoyed life. My childhood, teens and early twenties were all free of any major illnesses or problems. I had a real zest for life and enjoyed various social activities and sports, with a circle of friends. I have always been quite conscious about what I eat and tried to maintain a healthy diet, although not franatically, my only problem being an allergy to eggs (they gave me diarrhoea), and this developed in 1990. My career has spanned nursing, midwifery and health visiting, all of which I have enjoyed greatly, but all have their demand and stress factors; nonetheless, I enjoyed them. So when my illness was diagnosed it was a shock to everyone, including me.

Life was good. I had a boyfriend, a place of my own, good social life. Hence, when I had my bowels open one cold February morning and I passed bright red blood, I was extremely worried. Having seen my GP, I was then referred to a Consultant at the local hospital, who

218

I saw within 2 weeks. I underwent a sigmoidoscopy, which involved a tube being passed into the back passage to have a look at the bowel. From this uncomfortable experience, a diagnosis was made. In my case the diagnosis was ulcerative colitis. I felt numb, shocked, confused and bewildered. Physically, I was experiencing stomach cramps, diarrhoea and bleeding and did not feeling like eating. Surely a mistake had been made ... **why me!**

These were my initial thoughts, and even though I knew something about this debilitating disease from information learnt in my nurse training, it did little to ease my anxieties. After a chat with my consultant, my hope lay in the fact that I could be treated, with steroids and other medication and that it would only be a matter of time before I got better and my life would be back to normal. With this in mind, I tried to be positive and live with the illness. But alas the diarrhoea, bleeding and stomach pains persisted, and they culminated in a flare-up that would occur every 2-4 months, and I would have to increase the dose of steroids and take a couple of days off to deal with the excruciating pain and the debilitating effect it had on me. Along with the medication, I also tried complementary therapies, and as the years passed by I put up a fight against surgery and wanted to beat the disease on my own.

I knew in the back of my mind that, realistically I could not continue, and I tried to bring myself around to the thought of surgery. I sought information from a consultant at St Marks Hospital about the pouch surgery, and he had said I would be an ideal candidate, advising that this would be the best option **if** and **when** I decided. But I just could not face up to it, the thought of coping with major surgery and even more so with an ileostomy really scared me, but it was either surgery or a life of continuous steroids and medication with harmful side effects. I seemed to lose whichever way I turned.

In February 1996, I found myself in St Mark's Hospital with my life hanging in the balance, a weight of 6 stone, a tube down my nose to feed me a drip, and a needle in my arm for pain relief. I knew how I got there, but I do not know how it all happened. It is all somewhat of a blur, but my mind was so powerful and my body so weak, yet I had fought and fought until I could not go on any more and the surgeon's knife was my only reprieve.

My first operation was performed in February 1996 as an emergency to remove my diseased large bowel, which was causing me so much pain and had almost cost me my life. Because I had been so ill prior to surgery, it took me much longer to recover, and I spent three and a half months in hospital, after which I spent 2 weeks in a convalescence home, then the rest of my convalescence with my mother. In November 1996 I was ready for the second stage of surgery ... the formation of the pouch. Up until then, I had been building myself up in preparation, both physically and psychologically, for the next step. Recovery from the second operation took me some time, and because of this, the reversal was planned for April 1997.

So in total I had 14 months with an ileostomy. After the first few weeks of readjustment, and trying to generally cope, I discovered that I was dealing with the ileostomy much better than I had ever anticipated. That is not to say that I would have preferred to keep it, but by the end of the 14 months, I had got quite used to it. It went everywhere with me ... I never left home without it! However, I was so looking forward to having the ileostomy reversed and to sitting on the toilet to open my bowels and feeling 'normal' again.

In the first few days that followed the reversal of the ileostomy, the pouch was keeping me very busy. My trips to the toilet were between 10 and 15 times per day, and I was also getting up in the night. My bottom was really sore at times, and often after a trip to the toilet, after carefully washing and drying myself and applying cream, I would waddle back to my bed and lie on my side until the stinging and soreness had passed. Along with this, I had the occasional leak, which was sometimes distressing, but I had to believe that things would get better. I had come through so much in the 14 months, that I would come through this as well. The novelty of sitting on the toilet to have my bowels open normally (even though it was all liquid) took quite some time to wear off! It was a good feeling for me and another milestone in my recovery. I felt different without the ileostomy, and now I had to get used to the pouch, I remember looking down, expecting to see the bag, but it was no longer there and that did feel odd!

I was very cautious about what I ate and deep down had a real fear that I might block the pouch or cause it to function abnormally.

As the days passed, the pouch became more settled, and I became more confident with what I could eat. I found the first few weeks following the reversal quite exhausting, probably because I was so busy in the bathroom! I found that foods like banana, white rice and pasta helped to thicken the output of the pouch, whereas nuts, mushrooms and apples increased it. I also found that I became very thirsty, and I was encouraged to drink an electrolyte mix, as well as keep my fluid intake up. I still find this, and am quite aware of foods that I do not tolerate too well. It is a case of trial and error, but my diet and appetite have certainly improved, and my weight is back to normal.

This definitely varies from person to person, as I have had many conversations with other pouch owners and some have said they can eat virtually anything. For me, however, I had spent many years trying to control the colitis through diet so perhaps I have a psychological hangover on this. I am pleased that I am now able to enjoy a glass of wine, but if I have more that one glass the pouch becomes quite active. I also get anal irritation if I have eaten a meal with some spices in, especially black pepper. This can be quite uncomfortable, particularly if I am out and I long for the privacy of my own bathroom!

This leads me nicely onto the subject of **wind**! Yes, I did and do get terrible trapped wind, although it is much better now that I am more settled with eating. I find mint tea particularly good, and regular hot drinks. Sometimes the noises I make are quite loud, so the privacy of my own bathroom is a real plus. I do not have a problem with uncontrollable wind; my stomach may growl loudly when I am out, but I can usually make an excuse for that.

I had had such a build-up to all three operations, and had to be strong in between and all along the way, that when it was all over I did have a few days when I felt quite fed up. Over the past 14 months, I had gone through two major operations and a smaller one, I had been critically ill, experienced an ileostomy and I now had a pouch. I guess I was entitled to have a few 'off days'! It is a strange feeling to go from having an ileostomy to having a pouch; somehow I thought all my worries would be over and I could forget the surgery had ever happened. I thought that I could go back to using the toilet normally and everything would be OK again. If only things were so simple. Psychologically, I had flashbacks of the traumatic surgery and recovery. I still get these now but not as often. I not only have the emotional scars, but also the physical ones. Having an ileostomy made me really think about my body and what clothes I could wear in a way that I had never considered. Now that I have a pouch, I no longer have to wear baggy jumpers and loose T-shirts, and have reverted to close-fitting clothes.

Having said that, I still have the physical scar, and being intimate with my boyfriend was very difficult, plus the fact I felt different both inside my abdomen and inside my head! I did not want him to see my scars. I still had to get my head around them. I was also never very keen for him to see the ileostomy, although he did show a keen interest and he did see it once! My boyfriend (that was) was a good support to me all through the years of colitis, but our relationship suffered and we did split up earlier this year, not totally because of my illness and surgery but I feel that it played a significant part.

I am now 18 months post-reversal and am keeping very well, and the pouch is functioning well. I only need to empty it 4-5 times per day and do not get up in the night. However, I eat my main meal at lunchtime and I think this helps. Having a big meal late in the evening means I usually have to get up or I sometimes get a leak!

There is no urgency to get to the toilet; if I feel I have to go, I can always hang on for 1-2 hours. If I am going out or am away, I sometimes take loperamide tablets which slow down the pouch activity. At work, the pouch fits in well with my daily activities, and having good toilet facilities helps! I have a very active life with work, decorating my new home, visiting friends and family, writing and other social activities. I am also involved in a pouch support group in conjunction with the Ileostomy Association and am a member of the Red Lion Group. I do get extremely tired, but I know my limitations. I have had two episodes of pouchitis, for which I have taken Metronidazole tablets and it has resolved within a few days. It is not pleasant, but compared to the colitis it is manageable.

I have now left health visiting and I work as a clinical training officer; this job involves the teaching and training of qualified nurses. I have always enjoyed teaching, and this job is giving me the opportunity to develop my skills. I continue to eat well although I still need to avoid some foods such as nuts, mushrooms, cabbage and peppers, but in time I should be able to tolerate these.

The experience of colitis and surgery for me has spanned over 6 years, and at one stage I did not think I would live, but here I am writing about it in the hope that it will help others. I am delighted with the end result of all my surgery. The whole experience has been traumatic and the memories do not go away ... they only fade. I have been forced to re-focus on what is important in life, to filter out the trivialities and not take things for granted. A cliché but very true. The support from family, friends, colleagues and hospital staff has been invaluable. The pouch is working very well for me, I am colitis-free, and I have a good quality of life and my health is renewed. Long may it continue.

The pouch is an unknown quantity and if one day I have to revert to the ileostomy, then I will deal with it at that time. In the meantime, I intend to live life to the full!

Phil's story – Living with a Kock continent ileostomy

I'm 46 years old going on 10. Ulcerative colitis struck in 1992. I was immediately given medication to help combat this, which caused me numerous problems. As my condition deteriorated, I was prescribed a high dose of steroids, and reluctantly I gave this a try. Deterioration continued at an even faster pace, when finally it was suggested that the only way forward would be surgery.

I had a total colectomy and ileostomy in 1994. My health returned fairly immediately once I had recovered from the surgery, but I did not anticipate how this would me affect not only physically, but also mentally. Carrying out everyday things, however big or small, like playing with children and the dog, swimming or even working under the car made me wonder whether anyone would notice the bag or whether I would catch or tear the stoma on something.

The biggest problem that I found was when I looked into the mirror or when I wanted to take my T-shirt off in the hot weather. However much my wife and family supported me and tried to convince me that they were not affected by my appearance, the same feelings haunted me. I felt abnormal.

After the operation it was weird going to sleep and waking up with a thing (stoma) on your side and the pain, I remember the pain. At first I did not like looking at it (the stoma), the smell, the mess, what had I let them do to me? It had gone from one extreme to another, never requiring a hospital visit to this. Adjusting to the stoma and scars took time.

After having the ileostomy, my health had improved, and after 2 years of suffering my general health improved greatly. I continued to attend the hospital for outpatient appointments and soon began to discuss with the doctors the proposed reversal. I was able to discuss all my underlying fears. I was told that when I had fully recovered from this first operation, I would be able to have surgery that would connect me up as normal. I had to lose 2 stone before the surgery could be done. So no cream cakes for me! This was one of the hardest things I've had to do in my life, not mentioning the expense, going to the gym three or four times a week. The weight was lost, and in 1996 I was booked in to have the reversal surgery. Three days prior to the operation, an abscess formed in the area where the surgery was going to be performed. The muscles in my bottom where the re-connection was to occur had now been totally destroyed. All hopes had been destroyed. I was absolutely devastated at not being able to have the reconstruction surgery.

I spoke with my surgeon at great length and was offered an alternative form of surgery called a Kock pouch. Without much hesitation or discussing the implications fully I agreed to let him operate. What alternative did I have?

Once at home, I felt I did need more information. The stoma care nurse gave me an information booklet and also put me in touch with someone who had already had the operation. When I rang this person, he told me 'It's like converting from a Mini to Rolls Royce.' Enough said, I thought!

It was good to talk to someone because the nurses and doctors are only able to tell you so much. His words put me at ease. I know the main reason for going ahead with this surgery was vanity. Looking in a mirror with a bag stuck to your stomach was by no means a morale booster. I did, however, remember thinking was I making a big mistake; after all, since having the ileostomy my general health had been good. What risks was I undertaking? Could this be a mistake?

Before I knew it, the surgery was performed, there was no more decision-making, it just happened! The doctors and nurses were very supportive, and the stoma care nurse taught me how to use the catheter by inserting it into my pouch. It felt weird at first sticking a tube in the side of your stomach and watch the poo come out and go down the toilet. Sometimes it didn't come away easily so I was shown how to wash the pouch out with water.

The feeling of being bag-free was (and still is!) great. Having nothing visible around the waist line of my trousers, no risk of catching the bag and it tearing, no worry about odour. Carrying the catheter around is a small price to pay. I usually use a disabled toilet when I'm out and about. I've learnt that a normal toilet is not viable or practical. The difference that I found between the bag and the pouch is that you empty the bag when required, whereas you empty the pouch when it tells you.

My family feel that the illness has changed me, generally making me disgruntled. I can remember thinking, why me? What have I done wrong in life to deserve this? With time, I have begun to accept what has happened, and what will be will be. There are people who are worse off than me.

Most of my leisure time is taken up with DIY. This has included building a garden pond, renewing my kitchen, bricklaying, plastering, there is nothing that I will not attempt. When I have overdone things, my pouch will give me a warning.

In order to relax, I enjoy building and flying remote controlled aeroplanes. I enjoy a round of golf, but this has its drawbacks because a round usually takes 4-5 hours and there are no toilets at hand. I generally watch what I eat beforehand. I have started swimming again and enjoy it without having the embarrassment and worry of my appearance. My wildest of all hobbies is motorbikes. I own and ride a 900 cc motorbike for pure pleasure. Can anyone out there with a pouch beat my record of 130+mph; this must be the fastest pouch on earth!

I currently work for British Telecommunications and have done so for 25 years. They have accommodated to my needs in both a caring and a dignified manner. The overall support I received from managers and work colleagues, both at home and whilst in hospital, was overwhelming. Money is always a concern when you're ill, having been off for 3 months, I received full pay. I returned to work on a gradual basis until I felt confident.

My manager, in collaboration with the occupational health department, had made substantial changes in order for me to empty my pouch via the catheter in a safe, clean and dignified manner. The disabled toilet was totally refurbished, including a larger hand basin and a lockable cabinet for my equipment. Facilities had been made in the office area for easy access to refreshments, not only for me but also my colleagues.

To date, I have no regrets. I now feel I have adapted to the operation. I don't know how long the pouch will last, forever I hope, but then how long is ever?

Mary's story – Living with a continent urinary diversion

My name is Mary and I am at present 37 years old and work as a human resources manager for as restaurant company in Central London. I was born with no bladder, and at the age of 7, after many attempts, was given a urostomy at Great Ormond Street Hospital. Having learned to live with this tolerably well, at the age of 24 my consultant told me about an operation he was offering that would mean the removal of the dreaded urostomy and the chance of a relatively normal life. After thinking about it (for 5 minutes) I said 'Yes', not knowing that I was letting myself into a dreadful 6 months made bearable only by my mother, my friend (now my husband) Graham and some wonderful staff at the Shaftesbury Hospital.

My reasons for deciding to go for something new was that it would give me a chance at a more 'normal' life. I had never told any of my friends that I had a urostomy, and it made life very difficult in so many ways, especially as I got older. So the decision was not difficult to make, and if things really did not work out I could always go back to what I had before.

After four operations, the Kock pouch was in and working and I went home. This settling in period was difficult as I did not know what I was meant to feel physically and every little twinge and cramp meant something was collapsing - well, it did in my mind at least! There were also a few panics in the early days when the tube would not go in one especially memorable evening spent at the Shaftesbury Hospital following my engagement party! A couple of visits to my local casualty department and to the Shaftesbury were required before I was given a metal tube that acts as a sort of 'starter' if the catheter doesn't want to go in. This has proved to be very useful then and still is now, although it is only taken out a couple of times a year.

Another thing I found to worry about was the amount of 'gunk' (mucus) produced, but this seemed to clear up as time went on and did not cause a worry. At this time, I also felt that I had to be careful lifting and moving things as if I picked up something too heavy, I could certainly feel it! However, it was not too difficult for me to adapt, and the good things outweighed the bad. One aspect of the return to home that was difficult was that my GP was not knowledgeable about the operation I had gone through, so if I was worried I had to contact the hospital. This was OK at the beginning as I knew all the staff in the wards, but later on when the staff had changed, this was more difficult as I had no contact name.

Since having the Kock pouch, there are lots of things that have improved in my life. For instance, I had never been able to indulge myself and buy underwear or fitted clothes, so once I had recovered I had great fun buying new clothes that were fashionable. I gained confidence because I felt safer and more comfortable afterwards - no carrying around of spare bags and bits! There was no problem with smell any more and no nasty accidents, which had happened with a urostomy. And of course it's a lot nicer sleeping with someone without the extra bits attached!

Going on holiday was easier, and wearing a swimsuit wasn't such a scary experience any more - it was just fun. Staying at friends' homes had always been a bit of a trial, but it was a lot easier once I didn't have to hide in the bathroom for ages and carry supplies around 'just in case'. Although there were lots of things I could suddenly do, it was really overall confidence I gained because I felt more 'normal'. Those around me may not have seen a change but there was one.

Now onto the not-so-good bits, although I wouldn't say all of them are bad! One of the worst things has to be the higher incidence of urinary infections, which seems to be an ongoing problem.

However, with a little bit of thought and care, it is not so difficult except when I am feeling generally run down, tired or stressed, and those are the times it usually starts. As long as I remember to wash my hands before catheterizing, store the catheter properly and do wash-outs, the risk is reduced. Some things are also self-inflicted. For instance, leaving it too long to go the toilet can mean a very unpleasant pain that does not go away afterwards. If it is during the night or when I am very busy at work, I try to ignore the first twinges and hope it will go afterwards - it almost feels like it is bruised.

On a practical front, using public toilets (as opposed to your toilet at home) can cause a multitude of problems. Firstly you have to take a handbag everywhere, which is OK if you're female as that's fairly usual, although people do sometimes ask me why I'm taking my handbag to the toilet. My usual rejoinder is that it needs some exercise or something silly, which takes their mind off why they asked. The real fun starts once I have washed my hands and am in the cubicle. I store my catheter in a plastic bag, which has a plastic zip along the top. Great for storage but not for silence. Trying to open a plastic bag and take something out of it quietly is not easy. Then comes the bit where you can either make a decision not to make a noise when catheterizing or make lots of noise! Both sound strange to others because the former decision makes people wonder what you are doing, and the latter makes people wonder if you're odd because the way the urine comes out is much slower and takes longer!

Anyway once you've finished, you have to go out and wash and dry the catheter and then replace it in its bag. Not always possible if there are other people around. In order to avoid meeting others in the toilet, I try and choose quiet times such as the middle of the afternoon and not just before lunch or leaving times. A final note, the see-through plastic bags can cause an embarrassing incident if you open your bag forgetting that the last time you went to the toilet you just shoved it on the top of the things in your bag, not down the side as usual.

Another difficult situation can happen when you have been out for the evening and had a little bit too much to drink and have left it too long to go to the toilet. You eventually make it and find that the catheter does not want to play. As soon as this happens, you panic and this makes it even worse. The best way I have found to get round this is to stop thinking of what you are trying to do and just think of a totally unrelated subject. This takes your mind off what you are trying to do, which lets the muscles relax so that the catheter can go in - or that is certainly how it feels.

In retrospect, I feel that more information could have been given to me in a written form when I left hospital. I don't have a very good memory at the best of times, but when you are about to leave hospital after an extended stay of 4 months, four operations and a weight loss of a stone, whatever you are told disappears fast. I also feel that my GP could have given me more information on, for instance, post-hospital care and the use of wash-out etc. If the GP cannot be sent information directly, could the patient be given some written information to pass onto the GP for their file?

Looking at the amount I have written, the bad seems to outweigh the good, but my final comment would be that with all the little problems - and they are only little - I would not change back for anything. The last 12 years has been wonderful in giving me the freedom and confidence I always wanted and I would recommend it to anyone!

Caroline's story – Living with a colo-anal pouch

My name is Caroline; I am a 46-year-old mother of four and wife to Robert. We've been married for 25 years. My story begins back in 1995 when I started having bad diarrhoea. I went to see my GP, but the symptoms continued far about 6-8 months and I wasn't getting anywhere. I was initially treated for irritable bowel disease and given Imodium to try and control the diarrhoea.

Even though I was told I had irritable bowel, I knew I had cancer. I had all the symptoms that signify bowel cancer. Even though I was really concerned about this, my GP told me I was too young to have bowel cancer, and I got very depressed. Eventually, I sought a private opinion within a week was seen by a surgeon who told me I had a polyp. I did ask if this polyp could be cancerous, and they said definitely not. I had biopsies taken and bowel cancer was diagnosed. It didn't come as a surprise as I had lost so much weight. I had surgery followed by 1 year's treatment of a combination of radiotherapy and chemotherapy. I travelled into London for my treatment. I never felt unlucky to have cancer, just lucky that the cancer had been found and that I was having treatment for it.

I did get low in myself. I just plodded on for a couple of years and then the same symptoms returned: losing weight and constipation. Recent tests had been clear, but I pleaded and begged with the doctor to re-do the tests for me, which he agreed to do. I had more biopsies taken, which proved there was a recurrence of the cancer at the join of the bowel.

Because of the radiotherapy damage to the bowel, I was referred to St Mark's Hospital to see a specialist, who explained things to me. He explained to me about having a colo-anal pouch and put this forward as the best option for me. He then explained about having a temporary ileostomy. I was given some leaflets and was drawn a diagram of what the operation would be like.

Having the ileostomy gave me a new sense of freedom. I did things with the children I hadn't done in a long time. I went to the seaside for the first time in 2 years. It was great not to have to run to the toilet all the time. I was concerned about having the ileostomy reversed. I was warned about the size of the operation, but it proved to be a small one - I did have a few problems following this with blockages in the bowel. Some of it may have been what I was eating, but, I feel I would have benefited from more information from the dietitian.

I do feel positive about having the pouch. However, I do have to be careful what I eat or I can end up sitting on the toilet for most of the evening. I need to plan 24 hours in advance if I am going somewhere special to prevent having to go to the toilet a lot.

I'd like to get back to work again, but I know that whatever job I return to I will have to take care that there are toilet facilities readily available. I do feel my day-to-day activities are restricted, but I am also aware that my pouch is still settling into a pattern. I'll never be 100% normal again. A toilet being available is a constant worry. But it's great to be without a bag, without stomach pain and free from cancer.

I don't go out spontaneously; all events are planned in advance. I would like to get back to keep fit again, but the tiredness hasn't allowed me to do this yet. I have flown on a short flight and been to the theatre. I would recommend a pouch to anyone who asked for my opinion.

I don't find it easy to talk to people, and although I have been seen by Macmillan nurses I don't feel their role was explained to me properly. With regard to the pouch, I would have liked more information, especially on how long it would take for the pouch to settle. I have lost faith in some doctors and nurses, although I have found other medical staff very supportive.

I find it difficult to talk about the future: what I want to hear no-one can say. I want to hear that the cancer won't come back again.

Katy's story – Living with an ileo-anal pouch, a child's view

Writing this has been more difficult than I anticipated because it brought everything back to life. In one sense, it has been part of the healing process. I wasn't aware of the level of pain that had lain dormant within my being.

It all seems so long ago now, but 2 years ago I was thinking I had started my periods and was becoming a young woman, but in reality my body was telling me that something was terribly wrong. When you're 11 you don't really know your body very well, so how was I to know I was bleeding from the wrong place? Anyway, to cut a long story short, it became obvious that it wasn't my period, so I went to the doctor with my mum to see what it was.

When I was referred to the hospital for tests, I began to feel frightened and that everything was going out of my control. Having had many tests, I found the worst one was the sigmoidoscopy. Little did I know that I would need major surgery.

After the sigmoidoscopy, one of the doctors came to speak to me and told me that he had some bad news. That day I was diagnosed with polyposis. It was a very emotional day, not just for me, but also for my family. On the way home from hearing the news, I found my head was full with all sorts of things. I felt alone and afraid. There was so much anger in my heart, I just wanted to go to sleep in the hope that when I awoke; it would all have disappeared. But this was the reality; how could this disease just vanish from my body?

Because of the variety of the tests I had to have, I was referred to many hospitals. One hospital I did not particularly like because the specialist said to me that 'It didn't matter what I was going through, I could get over it.' Another thing which he said that stood out to me most was 'The Katy who comes in this hospital won't be the same Katy that goes home.' That really shocked me. How could a grown man with children of his own say something like this to a 12-year-old girl who really didn't understand what he was talking about? He told me that I had 'pre-cancerous cells on the polyps'. I couldn't believe it, cancer! I couldn't imagine how was I going to cope.

Then one day, my mum came across an article about a trial on a drug called FGN-1, which hoped to offer a cure for colon cancer. For days mum worked hard to find all the information that she could and even asked a neighbour in the medical world to surf the Internet for more details. From this, she spoke to people in America who were organizing the trials, and from there eventually to people in the Polyposis Registry at St Mark's hospital in London.

I was to have a second opinion at St Mark's. This time, I had to have a colonoscopy so I couldn't eat for a day. That was horrible! Afterwards, I spoke to a consultant who was very specific to me. He answered all my questions, which I really appreciate and he told me that apart from this situation, I was perfectly healthy, it was just my colon that was letting me down. He even said that I would still be the same Katy but that I wouldn't have my colon any more.

We decided that I would have my operation in London, and the date was booked. I had the operation at the end of September; it was really scary. I would never have thought that I would have to go through major surgery at the age of 13. Just before I went down to theatre, one of the doctors gave me a tablet to make me tired and to take the edge of things because I was really nervous. My mum and I had a little cry together; she didn't want her baby girl to go through this. Mum said I was really brave.

When I came out of theatre, I was in a lot of pain and I remember crying. Everyone said that I was doing really well, and I think I was for the first few days until day five. That was a bad day for me. I had been sick quite a lot and had lost a lot of weight. When I looked in the mirror, I couldn't see the real Katy. I looked so different. I hated my stoma. I was angry and wouldn't even touch it, but after talking to my mum, she helped me to see that 'this stoma', as she called it, had saved my life, and over the next few days I started to feel grateful to it rather than seeing it as my enemy. I had the odd day when I resented what had happened to me, but mum didn't let me stay down for long.

I stayed off school for weeks to recuperate. I think I adapted quite well to going back to school. I chose when to go to the toilet. At first, I kept to a strict diet, but a man who had a different disease but the same operation told me to eat what I wanted and ignore what happens afterwards, so I did. This helped me to start to regain the weight I had lost. I decided to have a feast at 11 o'clock at night, and I'm sure you can imagine what happened.

Five months after the first operation, I went back for the next step, which was the reversal of the stoma. This time I wasn't as scared because I couldn't wait to have it. At last it would be all over and I could be 'normal' once more. When I awoke from the operation this time, I was extremely cold and needed extra blankets and bedding. I could not believe I had reached this stage, needing only to get better in order to go home. For the first few days after the operation, I kept checking for the stoma, but of course it wasn't there. To this day, I can still feel some of the sensations I used to have with the stoma.

One of the reasons I came through this whole experience so well was that I had my family and friends with me, through both the good times and the bad. At times, I felt people did not know how to react around me - I think it concerned them more than me.

I have now seen my dad go through the same operation as me, even though I hated every single minute of it, it saved his life as well. Dad has now had both parts of the operation and is well on the road to recovery. When Dad had his stoma, he was very wary of what to eat and drink. I said to him, 'Dad get a life! Eat what you fancy and don't worry too much about it.'

Polyposis is familial, which means it can be passed down from generation to generation, and my brother and three sisters went through tests to see if they had the same genes as my Dad and me. Fortunately, only my younger sister was found to be positive but she will wait until my age before we think about any operation. What we do know is that she will have the same support that my dad and me had.

Now it is all over, I am back at school living a normal life and have put it all behind me.

Useful addresses

British Association for Counselling
1 Regent Place
Rugby
Warwickshire CV21 2PJ
(01788) 550899
www.counselling.co.uk

British Colostomy Association (BCA)
15 Station Road
Reading
Berkshire RG1 1LG
(0118) 939 1537
www.bcass.org.uk

CancerBACUP
3 Bath Place
Rivington Street
London EC2A 3JR
020 7613 2121 or 0808 800 1234

Cancer Care Society
Jane Scarth House
39 The Hundred
Romsey
Hampshire SO51 8GE
(01794) 830374

Cancerlink
11–21 Northdown Street
London N1 9BN
020 7840 7840

Colon Cancer Concern
4 Rickett Street
London SW6 1RU
020 7381 4711

Continence Foundation
307 Hatton Square
16 Baldwins Gardens
London EC1N 7RJ
020 7404 6875
www.continence-foundation.org.uk

Crohn's in Childhood Research Association (CICRA)
Parkgate House
356 West Barnes Lane
Motspur Park
Surrey KT3 6NB
020 8949 6209
support@cicra.org
www.cicra.org.

Family Fund Trust
PO Box 50
York YO1 2ZX

Ileostomy and Internal Pouch Support Group (ia)
PO Box 132
Scunthorpe
North Lincolnshire DN15 9YW
(01724) 720150
www.ileostomypouch.demon.co.uk

Impotence Association
PO Box 10296
London SW17 9WH
020 8767 7791

Macmillan Cancer Relief
Anchor House
15/19 Britten Street
London SW3 3TZ
020 7351 7811 or 0845 601 6161

National Advisory Service for the Parents of Children with a Stoma
51 Anderson Drive
Darvel
Ayrshire KA17 0DE
(01560) 322024

National Association of Crohn's and Colitis (NACC)
PO Box 205
St Albans,
Hertfordshire AL1 1AB
(01727) 844296 Fax (01727) 862550
www.nacc.org.uk

Network 81
1–7 Woodfield Terrace
Stansted
Essex CM24 8AJ
(01279) 647415 Fax (01279) 814908

Red Lion Group
Liaison Officer
c/o St Mark's Hospital
Watford Road
Harrow
Middlesex HA1 3UJ
020 8235 4126
www.red-lion-group.mcmail.com

Royal Association for Disability and Rehabilitation (RADAR)
12 City Forum
250 City Road
London EC1V 8AF
020 7250 3222

St Mark's Polyposis Registry
Helpline 020 8235 4270

Smilie's People
5 Laws Close
Milking Nook
Peterborough
Northamptonshire PE6 7PS
(01733) 810413

Urostomy Association (UA)
Buckland
Beaumont Park
Danbury
Essex CM3 4DE
(01245) 224294

References

Ament ME, Berquist M, Vargas J (1988) Advances in ulcerative colitis. Pediatrician 15(1–2): 45–57.

Atkin W, Cuzick J, Northover JMA, Whynes D (1993) Prevention of colorectal cancer by once-only sigmoidoscopy. Lancet 341: 736–40.

Avorn J, Monane M, Gurwitz JH, Glynn RJ et al (1994) Reduction of bacteruria and pyuria after ingestion of cranberry juice. Journal of the American Medical Association 271(10): 751–4.

Awad RW, el-Gohary TM, Skilton JS, Elder JB (1993) Life quality and psychological morbidity with an ileostomy. British Journal of Surgery 80(2): 252–3.

Aylett SO (1953) Conservative surgery in the treatment of ulcerative colitis. British Medical Journal 2: 1348–51.

Aylett SO (1966) Three hundred cases of diffuse ulcerative colitis treated by total colectomy and ileo-rectal anastomosis. British Medical Journal i: 1001–5.

Baider L, Koch U, Esacson R, Kaplan de-Noir (1998) Prospective study of cancer patients and their spouses: the weakness of marital strength. Psycho-Oncology 7: 49–56.

Bain IM, Mostafa AB, Harding LK, Neoptolemos JP, Keighley MRB (1995) Bile acid absorption from ileoanal pouches using enema scintigraphy. British Journal of Surgery 82: 614–17.

Baker WNW, Glass RE, Ritchie JK, Alyett SO (1978) Cancer of the rectum following colectomy and ileorectal anastomosis for ulcerative colitis. British Journal of Surgery 65: 862–8.

Bambrick M, Fazio V, Hull T, Pucel G (1996) Sexual functioning following restorative proctocolectomy in women. Diseases of the Colon and Rectum 39: 610–14.

Batchelor D, Grahn G, Oliver G, Pritchard P, Redmond K, Webb P (1991) Cancer Care – Priorities for Nurses (Altered Body Image). European Oncology Nursing Society.

Becker J et al (1991) Late functional adaptation after colectomy, mucosal proctectomy and ileal pouch–anal anastomosis. Surgery 110(4): 718–24, discussion 725.

Beitz J (1999) The lived experience of having an ileoanal reservoir: a phenomenologic study. Journal of Wound, Ostomy and Continence Nursing 26(4): 185–200.

Belliveau P, Trudel J, Vasilevsky CA, Stein B, Gordon PH (1999) Ileoanal anastomosis with reservoirs: complications and long-term results. Canadian Journal of Surgery 42(5): 345–52.

Berger A, Tiret E, Parc R (1992) Excision of the rectum with colonic J pouch–anal anastomosis for adenocarcinoma of the low and mid rectum. World Journal of Surgery 16(3): 470–7.

Berk T, Cohen Z, Mcleod RS, Stern HS (1992) Management of mesenteric desmoid tumours in F.A.P. Canadian Journal of Surgery 35(4): 393.

Black P (1997) Familial Adenomatous Polyposis. Eurostoma 18: 8–9.

Blackmore C (1988) The oncological perspective. In Salter M (Ed) Altered Body Image – the Nurse's Role. Chichester: John Wiley.

Bleeker H, Mulderij K (1992) The experience of motor disability. Phenomenology and Pedagogy 10: 1–18.

Bodmer WF et al (1987) Localization of the gene for familial adenomatous polyposis on chromosome 5. Nature 328: 614–162.

Bond C, Bailey B, Corry D, Jones D, Notter J (1997) A survey of patients' perceptions of life with an ileo-anal pouch. British Journal of Community Health Nursing 2(1): 52–8.

Bond S (1997) Eating Matters: A Resource for Improving Dietary Care in Hospitals. Newcastle: University of Newcastle Centre for Health Services Research.

Borwell B (1997) Ileo-anal pouch surgery and its after-care. Community Nurse 3(7): 15020.

Borwell B (1998) Developing Sexual Helping Skills: A Guide for Nurses. Maidenhead: Medical Projects.

Brandberg A, Kock NG, Phillipson B (1972) Bacterial flora in intraabdominal ileostomy reservoir. A study of 23 patients provided with 'continent ileostomy'. Gasteroenterology 63: 413–16.

Brevinge H, Berglund B, Kock NG (1992a) Ileostomy output of gas and faeces before and after conversion from conventional to reservoir ileostomy. Diseases of the Colon and Rectum 35: 662–9.

Brevinge H, Bosaeus I, Philipson BM, Kewenter J (1992b) Sodium and potassium excretion before and after conversion from conventional to reservoir ileostomy. International Journal of Colorectal Disease 7: 148–54.

Bricker EM (1950) Bladder substitution after pelvic evisceration. Surgical Clinics of North America 30: 1151.

Bronner C, Baker S, Morrison P (1994) Mutation in the DNA mismatch repair gene homologue hMLH1 is associated with heredity non-polyposis colon cancer. Nature 368: 258–61.

Brooke BN (1952) The management of ileostomy. Lancet ii: 102–4.

Brydolf M (1996) Living with ulcerative colitis. Journal of Advanced Nursing 23(1): 39–47.

Buess G, Mentges B, Mannke K (1992) Technique and results of transanal endoscopic microsurgery in early rectal cancer. American Journal of Surgery 163: 63–70.

Buller HA (1997) Problems in diagnosis of IBD in children. Netherlands Journal of Medicine 50(2): 8–11.

Burnard J, Morrison L (1990) Body image and physical appearance. Surgical Nurse 3: 4–8.

Burnham W, Lennard-Jones J, Brooke B (1977) Sexual problems amongst married ileostomists. Gut 18: 673–7.

Bussey H (1975) Familial Polyposis Coli. Family Studies, Histopathology, Differential Diagnosis and Results of Treatment. Johns Hopkins University Press.

Cameron K, Gregor F (1987) Chronic illness and compliance. Journal of Advanced Nursing 12: 671–6.

Carapeti EA, Kamm MA, Evans BK, Phillips RKSP (1999) Topical phenylephrine increases anal sphincter resting pressure. British Journal of Surgery 86: 267–70.

Carolan C (1984) Sex and disability. Nursing Times 80(39): 28–30.

Caven A (1996) Introducing The Family Fund Trust. York: York Publishing Services.

Chartrand-Lefebvre C, Heppell J, Davignon I, Dubè S, Pomp A (1990) Dietary habits after ileal pouch-anal anastomosis. Canadian Journal of Surgery 33: 101–5.

Chester J and Britton D (1989) Elective and emergency surgery for colorectal cancer in a district general hospital: impact of surgical training on patient survival. Annals of the Royal College of Surgeons of England 71: 370–4.

Christie PM, Knight GS, Hill GL (1990) Metabolism of body water and electrolytes after surgery for ulcerative colitis: conventional ileostomy versus J pouch. British Journal of Surgery 77: 149–51.

Christie PM, Knight GS, Hill GL (1996) Comparison of relative risks of urinary stone formation after surgery for ulcerative colitis: conventional ileostomy vs. J-pouch. Diseases of the Colon and Rectum 39: 50–4.

Chu K, Tarone R, Chow W, Hankey B, Riles L (1994) Temporal patterns in colorectal cancer incidence, survival and mortality form 1950 through 1990. Journal of the National Cancer Institute 86: 997–1006.

Church J (1986) The current status of the Kock continent ileostomy. Ostomy/Wound Management (Spring): 32–5.

Cochrane J, Faber R (1995) Value of outpatient follow-up after curative surgery for carcinoma of the large bowel. British Medical Journal 280: 593–5.

Coffey RC (1911) Physiologic implantation of the severed ureter or common bile duct into the intestine. Journal of American Medical Association 5: 97–403.

Cohen A (1991) Body image in the person with a stoma. Journal of Enterostomal Therapy 18(2): 14–16.

Cohen F, Lazarus RS (1982) Active coping processes, coping dispositions and recovery from surgery. Psychosomatic Medicine 35: 375–89.

Cohen Z (1985) The pelvic pouch and ileoanal anastomosis procedure. Surgical technique and initial results. American Journal of Surgery 150(5): 601–7.

Coran AG (1990) A personal experience with 100 consecutive total colectomies and straight ileoanal endorectal pull-through for benign disease of the colon and rectum in children and adults. Annals of Surgery 212(3): 242–7.

Corner J (1998) Nursing as a therapy. Paper presented on 9 February, Royal Marsden NHS Trust.

Cranley B (1983) The Kock reservoir ileostomy: a review of its development, problems and role in modern surgical practice. British Journal of Surgery 70: 94–9.

Crosland A, Jones R (1995) Rectal bleeding: prevalence and consultation behaviour. British Medical Journal 311: 486–8.

Curless R, French J, Williams G, James O (1994) Comparison of gastrointestinal symptoms in colorectal carcinoma patients and community controls with respect to age. Gut 35: 1267–70.

Curtis RD, Sweeney WB, Denobile JW, Hurwitz E (1996) Kock pouch dysfunction during pregnancy – management of a case. Surgical Endoscopy 10: 755–7.

Darbyshire P (1986) Body image – when the face doesn't fit. Nursing Times 24: 28–30.

Davis C, Alexander F, Lavery I, Fazio VW (1994) Results of mucosal proctectomy versus extrarectal dissection for ulcerative colitis and familial polyposis in children and young adults. Journal of Paediatric Surgery 29: 305–9.

Department of Health (1991) Welfare of Children and Young People in Hospital. London: HMSO.

DeSilva HJ, Mortensen NJ (1992) Persistent ileitis after salvage from a failed Kock pouch. Journal of Gastroenterology and Hepatology 7: 367–9.

Desparmet J, Desmazs N, Mazait X, Ecoffey C (1990) Evolution of regional anaesthesia in a paediatric surgical practice. In Tyler DC, Krone EJ (Eds) Advances in Pain Research Therapy. New York: Raven Press.

Devlin H, Plant J, Griffin M (1971) Aftermath of surgery for ano-rectal cancer. British Medical Journal 3: 413–18.

Dixon C (1939) Surgical removal of lesions occurring in the sigmoid and rectosigmoid. American Journal of Surgery 46: 12–17.

Dozois R, Kelly K, Beart R Jr et al (1980) Improved results with continent ileostomy. Annals of Surgery 192: 319–24.

Dozois RR, Goldberg SM, Rothenburger DA et al (1986) Restorative proctocolectomy with ileal reservoir. International Journal of Colorectal Disease 1(2): 19.

Druss R, O'Connor J, Prudden J, Sten L (1968) Psychologic response to colectomy. Archives of General Psychiatry 18: 53–9.

Dudley HAF (1978) If I had carcinoma of the middle third of the rectum. British Medical Journal l: 1035–67.

Dukes C (1929) The spread of cancer of the rectum. British Journal of Surgery 17: 643–8.

Dukes CE (1958) Cancer control in familial polyposis of the colon. Diseases of the Colon and Rectum 1: 412–23.

Dunkel-Schetter C (1984) Social support and cancer: Findings based on patient interviews and their implications. Journal of Social Issues 40: 77–98.

Durno C, Sherman P, Harris K et al (1998) Outcome after ileoanal anastomosis in paediatric patients with ulcerative colitis. Journal of Paediatric Gastroenterology and Nutrition 27(5): 501–7.

Dyk RB, Sutherland AM (1956) Adaptation of the spouse and other family to the colostomy patient. Cancer 9: 123–38.

Eardley A, Geroge W, Davis F et al (1976) Colostomy – the consequences of surgery. Clinical Oncology 2: 277–83.

Eccles DM (1997) An unusually severe phenotype for familial adenomatous polyposis. Archives of Diseases in Childhood 77(5): 431–5.

Ecker KW, Hildebrandt U, Haberer M, Feifel G (1996) Biochemical stabilization of the nipple valve in continent ileostomy. British Journal of Surgery 83: 1582–5.

Eckhoff DE, Starling JR, Anderson AB, Harms BA (1994) Proctocolectomy and quadruple-limb W pouch reconstruction for the management of paediatric ulcerative colitis and familial polyposis. Journal of Paediatric Surgery 29: 504–9.

Ell KO, Mantell JE, Hamovitch MB, Nishimoto RH (1989) Social support, sense of control, and coping among patients with breast, lung, or colorectal cancer. Journal of Psychosocial Oncology 7(3): 63–89.

Englert G, Hass M (1986) Patient's experience with the Kock pouch. Ostomy International (Dec): 10–12.

Erwin-Toth P (1999) The effect of ostomy surgery between the ages of 6 and 12 years on psychosocial development during childhood, adolescence and young adulthood. Journal of Wound, Ostomy and Continence Nursing 26(2): 77–85.

Erwin-Toth P, Spencer M (1991) A survey of patient perception of quality of care. Journal of Enterostomal Therapy Nursing 18(4): 122–5.

Evans BD (1995) The experiences and needs of patients attending a cancer support group. International Journal of Palliative Care 1(4): 189–94.

Everett W (1989) Restorative procto-colectomy with ileal reservoir. British Journal of Surgery 16(1): 77–81.

Faller MC, Welling RE, Lambert CE (1986) Nutritional implications and dietary management postproctocolectomy and ileal reservoir construction. Journal of the American Dietetic Association 86: 1235–6.

Farrelly R (1994) The special care needs of adolescents in hospital. Nursing Times 90(38): 31.

Fazio V (1995) Ileal pouch–anal anastomoses, complications and function in 1005 patients. Annals of Surgery 222(2): 120–7.

Fazio VW, Church JM (1988) Complications and function of the continent ileostomy at the Cleveland Clinic. World Journal of Surgery 12: 148–54.

Fazio V, Ziv Y, Church J et al (1995) Ileo pouch–anal anastomoses complications and function in 1005 patients. Annals of Surgery 222: 120–7.

Fearson E, Vogelstein B (1990) A genetic modal for colorectal tumorigenesis. Cell 61: 759–67.

Fillingham S (1997) Urological Stomas. In Fillingham S, Douglas J (Eds) Urological Nursing, 2nd Edn. London: Baillière Tindall.

Fiorentini MT, Locatelli L, Ceccopieri B et al (1987) Physiology of ileoanal anastomosis with ileal reservoir for ulcerative colitis and adenomatosis coli. Diseases of the Colon and Rectum 30: 267–72.

Fisch M, Hohenfellner R (1991) Der Sigma rektum pouch: eine modifikation der harnleiterdarm implantation. Aktuelle Urologie 22 Operative Techniken.

Fisch M, Wammeck R, Hohenfellner R (1992) The sigma-rectum pouch (Mainz pouch II). In Hohnefellner R, Wammeck R (Eds) Societé Internationale D'Urologie reports: Continent Urinary Diversion. Edinburgh: Churchill Livingstone.

Fitjen G, Starmans R, Muris J, Schouten H, Blijhaus G, Kuttinerus J (1995) Predictive value of signs and symptoms for colorectal cancer in patients with rectal bleeding in general practice. Family Practice 12: 279–86.

Fonkalsrud EW, Loar N (1992) Long-term results after colectomy and endorectal ileal pull-through procedure in children. Annals of Surgery 215(1): 57–62.

Frizelle FA, Burt MJ (1997) The surgical management of ulcerative colitis. Journal of Gastroenterology and Hepatology 12: 670–7.

Fuchs KH, Sailer M, Kraemer M, Thiede A (1998) Coloanal J-pouch reconstruction following low rectal resection. Recent Results in Cancer Research 146: 87–94.

Fujita S, Kusunoki M, Shoji Y, Owada T, Utsonomiya J (1992) Quality of life after total proctocolectomy and ileal J-pouch-anal anastomosis. Diseases of the Colon and Rectum 1135: 1030–9.

Gadacz TR, Kelly KA, Phillips SF (1997) The continent ileal pouch: absorptive and motor features. Gastroenterolgy 72: 1287–91.

Gage T (1986) Managing the cancer risk in chronic ulcerative colitis. Journal of Clinical Gastroenterology 8: 50–7.

Gerber A, Malcolm K, Apt MD, Craig PH (1983) The improved quality of life with the Kock continent ileostomy. Journal of Clinical Gastroenterology 6: 513–17.

Gerhardsson-de-Verdier M, Hagman U, Peters R (1991) Meat, cooking methods and colorectal cancer: a case referent study in Stockholm. International Journal of Cancer 49: 520–5.

Go PM, Lens J, Bosman FT (1987) Mucosal alterations in the reservoir of patients with Kock's continent ileostomy. Scandinavian Journal of Gastroenterology 22: 1076–80.

Goffman E (1963) Notes on the Management of Spoiled Identity. Prentice Hall: New York.

Goldberg SM (1987) Proctocolectomy and ileoanal anastomosis with an S pouch: functional results. Canadian Journal of Surgery 30: 359–61.

Golligher J (1983) Alternatives to conventional ileostomy in the surgical treatment of ulcerative colitis. Journal of Enterostomal Therapy 10: 79–83.

Gottlieb MD, Jacob C, Handelsman MD (1991) Treatment of outflow tract problems associated with continent ileostomy (Kock pouch). Diseases of the Colon and Rectum 34: 936–40.

Goulston K (1980) Role of diet in screening with fecal occult blod tests. Colorectal Cancer: Prevention, Epidemiology and Screening 271–4.

Goulston K, Dent O (1986) How important is rectal bleeding in the diagnosis of bowel cancer or polyps? Lancet i: 261–5.

Graf W, Dahlberg M, Ohlberg M, Holmberg L, Pahlman L, Glimelius B (1997) Short term pre-operative radiotherapy results in down staging of rectal cancer: a study of 1316 patients. Radiotherapy and Oncology 43: 133–7.

Greegor D (1971) Occult blood testing for detection of asymptomatic colon cancer. Cancer 28: 131–3.

Grobler S, Hosie K, Keighly M (1992) Randomised trial of loop ileostomy in restorative proctocoletomy. British Journal of Surgery 79: 903–6.

Groom S, Kamm MA, Nicholls RJ (1994) Relationship of small bowel motility and ileoanal reservoir function. Gut 35: 523–9.

Guerrero D (1997) Neuro-oncology for Nurses. London: Whurr.

Guillebaud J (1993) Contraception. Your Questions Answered, 2nd Edn. Churchill Livingstone, Edinburgh.

Gutman M, Fidler I (1995) Biology of human colon cancer metastasis. World Journal of Surgery 19: 226–34.

Hallbrook O, Pahlman L, Krog M, Wexner SD, Sjodahl R (1996) Randomized comparison of straight and colonic J pouch after low anterior resection. Annals of Surgery 224(1): 58–65.

Hamilton S (1996) Prevention and early diagnosis of colorectal cancer. R.A.L. Young, London: W.B. Saunders.

Hammer E (1929) Cancer du colon sigmoide dix ans après implantation des uretère d'une vessie exstrophiée. Journal d'Urologie 28: 260.

Hampton BG, Bryant RA (1992) Ostomies and continent diversions – nursing management. Missouri: Mosby Year Book.

Handelsman MD, Gottlieb MD, Stanley R, Hamilton MD (1993) Crohn's disease as a contraindication to Kock pouch (continent ileostomy). Diseases of the Colon and Rectum 36: 840–3.

Hardcastle J, Chamberlain JO, Robinson MH (1996) Randomised trial of faecal occult blood screening for colorectal cancer. Lancet 348: 1472–7.

Harter S (1982) The perceived competence scale for children. Child Development 53: 87–97.

Harvey PR, McLeod RS, Cohen Z, Strasberg SM (1991) Effect of colectomy on bile composition, cholesterol crystal formation, and gallstones in patients with ulcerative colitis. Annals of Surgery 214: 396–401.

Haward R (1997) Improving outcomes in colorectal cancer. The Manual, NHS Executive.

Hawley PR (1988) Emergency surgery for ulcerative colitis. World Journal of Surgery 12: 169–73.

Heald R, Karanjia N (1992) Results of radical surgery for rectal cancer. World Journal of Surgery 16: 848–57.

Heald R, Ryall R (1986) Recurrence and survival after total mesorectal excision for rectal cancer. Lancet 1: 1479–82.

Health Education Authority (1996) The Balance of Good Health. Marston Book Services.

Hendrick J (1997) Consent to treatment. In Legal Aspects of Child Health Care. London: Chapman & Hall.

Heppel J, Kelly KA, Phillips SF, Beart RW, Telander RL, Perrault J (1982) Physiologic aspects of continence after colectomy, mucosal proctectomy and endorectal ileo-anal anastomosis. Annals of Surgery 195: 435–43.

Hildebrandt U, Feifel G (1995) Preoperative staging of rectal cancer by intrarectal ultrasound. Diseases of the Colon and Rectum 28: 42–6.

Ho YH, Tan M, Seow-Choen F (1996) Prospective randomized controlled study of clinical function and anorectal physiology after low anterior resection: comparison of straight and colonic J pouch anastomosis. British Journal of Surgery 83(7): 978–80.

Hodgson SV, Bishop DT, Dunlop MG, Evans DG, Northover JMA (1995) Suggested screening guidelines for familial colorectal cancer. Journal of Medical Screening 2(1): 45–51.

Hoffenberg EJ, Sanaia A, Maltzman T, Knoll K, Ahnen DJ (1999) Symptomatic colonic polyps in childhood: not so benign. Journal of Paediatric Gastroenterology and Nutrition 28(2): 175–81.

Hojlund Pederson B, Simonson L, Kuld Hansen L et al (1985) Bile acid malabsorption in patients with an ileum reservoir with a long efferent leg to an anal anastomosis. Scandinavian Journal of Gastroenterology 20: 995–1000.

Hojo K, Sawada T, Moriya Y (1989) An analysis of survival and voiding, sexual function after wide ileopelvic lymphadenectomy in patients with carcinoma of the rectum, compared with conventional lymphadenectomy. Diseases of the Colon and Rectum 32: 128–33.

Holliday H, Hardcastle J (1979) Delay in diagnosis and treatment of symptomatic colorectal cancer. Lancet: 309–311.

Horowitz M (1966) Body Image. Archives of General Psychiatry 14: 213–20.

Hoyman K, Rolstad B (1992) Continent diversions and reservoirs. In Hampton B, Bryant R (Eds). Ostomies and Continent Diversions. St Louis: Mosby-Year Book.

Hughes A (1991) Life with a stoma. Nursing Times 87(25): 67–8.

Hughes KS, Rosenstein RB, Songhora bodi S (1988) Resection of the liver for colorectal carcinoma metastases. A multi-institutional study of long-term survivors. Diseases of the Colon and Rectum 31(1): 1–4.

Hull T (1999) Ileoanal procedures: acute and long-term management issues. Journal of Wound, Ostomy and Continence Nursing 26(4): 201–6.

Hull TL, Erwin-Toth P (1996) The pelvic pouch procedure and continent ostomies: overview and controversies. Journal of Wound, Ostomy and Continence Nursing 23: 156–65.

Hulten L, Fasth S, Nordgren S, Oresland T (1988) Kock's pouch converted to a pelvic pouch, a case report. Diseases of the Colon and Rectum 31: 467–9.

Hyams S (1996) Goodbye Stromboli... Journal 154: 16–17.

Hylander E, Ladefoged K, Lykkegaard Nielsen M, Vagn Nielsen O, Thale M, Jarnum S (1986) Excretion, deconjugation, and absorption of bile acids after colectomy for ulcerative colitis. Comparative studies in patients with conventional ileostomy and patients with Kock's reservoir. Scandinavian Journal of Gastroenterology 21: 1137–43.

Hylander E, Rannem T, Hegnhoj J, Kirkegarrd P, Thale M, Jarnum S (1991) Absorption studies after ileal J-pouch anastomosis for ulcerative colitis. A prospective study. Scandinavian Journal of Gastroenterology 26: 65–72.

Hyman NH, Fazio VW, Tuckson WB, Lavery IC (1991) Consequences of ileal pouch–anal anastomosis for Crohn's colitis. Diseases of the Colon and Rectum 34: 653–7.

Jackson WD, Grand RJ (1991) Crohn's disease. Paediatric Gastrointestinal Disease.

Jagenburg R, Kock NG, Philipson B (1975) Vitamin B12 absorption in patients with continent ileostomy. Scandinavian Journal of Gastroenterology 10: 141–4.

Jass JR, Love B, Northover JMA (1987) A new prognostic classification of rectal cancer. Lancet 1(8545): 1303–6.

Johnston D, Holdsworth PJ, Nasmyth DG et al (1987) Preservation of the entire anal canal in conservative proctocolectomy for ulcerative colitis: a pilot study. British Journal of Surgery 74: 940–4.

Jorge JMN, Wexner SD, James K, Nogueras JJ, Jagelman DG (1994) Recovery of anal sphincter function after the ileoanal reservoir procedure in patients over the age of fifty. Diseases of the Colon and Rectum 37: 1002–5.

Karthenser AH and others (1996) Ileal pouch-anal anastomosis as the first choice operation in patients with FAP: a ten year experience. Surgery 119(6): 615–23.

Keighley M (1990) The Pelvic Pouch: Restorative Proctocolectomy and Reservoir Ileoanal Anastomosis: Twenty Questions. Birmingham: Gastroenterological Units of the General and Queen Elizabeth Hospitals.

Keighley MRB (1996) Review: the management of pouchitis. Alimentary Pharmacology and Therapeutics 10: 449–57.

Keighley MRB, Williams NS (1993) Surgery of the anus, rectum and colon. London: WB Saunders.

Keighley MRB, Winslet MC, Pringle W, Allan RN (1987) The pouch as an alternative to permanent ileostomy. British Journal of Hospital Medicine (Oct): 287–92.

Keighley MRB, Grobler S, Bain I (1993) An audit of restorative proctocolectomy. Gut 34: 680–4.

Kenney RM (1986) Conventional versus continent ileostomy. WCET Journal (Nov): 13.

Killingback M (1985) Local excision for colorectal cancer: indications for local excision of rectal cancer. British Journal of Surgery Suppl: S54-S56.

King DW, Lubrowski DZ, Cook TA (1989) Anal canal mucosa in restorative proctocolectomy for ulcerative colitis. British Journal of Surgery 76: 970–2.

Kock NG (1969) Inter-abdominal 'reservoir' in patients with permanent ileostomy: preliminary observations on a procedure resulting in faecal continence in 5 ileostomy patients. Archives of Surgery 99: 223–31.

Kock NG (1992) The evolution of the urinary bladder. In Hohenfellner R, Wammeck R (Eds) Societé Internationale d' Urologie Reports: Continent Urinary Diversion. Edinburgh: Churchill Livingstone.

Kohler L, Troidl H (1995) The ileoanal pouch a risk–benefit analysis. British Journal of Surgery 82(4): 443–7.

Kohler L, Pemberton J, Zinsmeister A, Kelly A (1991) Quality of life after proctocolectomy. A comparison of Brooke ileostomy, Kock pouch and ileal pouch–anal anastomosis. Gastroenterology 101(3): 679–84.

Kohler LW, Pemberton JH, Hodge DO, Zinsmeister AR, Kelly KA (1992) Long term functional results and quality of life after ileal pouch–anal anastomosis and cholecystectomy. World Journal of Surgery 6(16): 1126–31.

Krook J, Moertel CG, Gunderson LL (1991) Effective adjuvant therapy for high-risk rectal carcinoma. New England Journal of Medicine 324: 709–15.

Kuhbacher T, Schreiber S, Runkel N (1998) Pouchitis: pathophysiology and treatment. International Journal of Colorectal Disease 13(5–6): 196–207.

Kuykendall J (1988) Teenage trauma. Nursing Times 85(27): 26–8.

Lackner S, Goldenberg S, Arizza G, Tjoswold I (1994) The contingency of social support. Qualitative Health Research 4(2): 224–43.

Lapides J, Diokno AC, Silber SJ, Lowe BS (1972) Clean intermittent self-catheterisation in the treatment of urinary tract disease. Journal of Urology 107: 458–61.

Leaver RB (1994) The Mitrofanoff pouch: a continent urinary diversion. Professional Nurse 9(11): 748–53.

Leaver R (1996a) Cranberry juice. Professional Nurse (May 8): 525–6.

Leaver RB (1996b) Continent urinary diversions – the Mitrofanoff principle. In Myers C (Ed) Stoma Care Nursing: A Patient-Centred Approach. London: Arnold.

Leaver RB (1997) Reconstructive surgery for the promotion of continence. In Fillingham S, Douglas J (Eds) Urological Nursing. London: Baillière Tindall/Royal College of Nursing.

Leaver RB (1998) Living with a Continent Urinary Diversion: A Qualitative Study of the Effects on Quality of Life of Patients. Unpublished dissertation.

Lennard-Jones JE (1991) Coping with the short bowel. Hospital Update (Oct): 797–807.

Lennard-Jones JE (1994) Review article: practical management of the short bowel. Alimentary Pharmacology and Therapeutics 8: 563–77.

Leppert M, Dobbs P, Scambler P, O'Connell SD, Nakamura Y et al (1987) The gene for familial polyposis coli maps to the long arm of chromosome 5. Science 238: 1411–13.

Lerch MM, Braun J, Harder M, Hofstadter F, Schumpelick V, Matern S (1989) Postoperative adaptation of the small intestine after total colectomy and J-pouch-anal anastomosis. Diseases of the Colon and Rectum 32: 600–8.

Levitt MD, Kuan M (1998) The physiology of ileo-anal pouch function. American Journal of Surgery 176: 384–9.

Levitt MD, Kamm MA, Nicholls RJ (1991) Pouch dynamics – a simple test of ileo-anal pouch evacuation. International Journal of Colorectal Diseases 6: 158–60.

Lewis WG, Sagar PM, Holdsworth PJ, Axon AT, Johnston D (1993) Restorative procto-colectomy with end to end pouch–anal anastomosis in patients over the age of fifty. Gut 34(7): 948–52.

Lieberman D, Smith S (1991) Screening for colonic malignancy with colonoscopy. American Journal of Gastroenterology 86: 946–51.

Loeschke K, Bolkert T, Kiefhaber P, Ruckdeschel G (1980) Bacterial overgrowth in ileal reservoirs (Kock pouch): extended functional studies. Hepto-Gastroenterology 27: 310–16.

Lohmuller JL, Pemberton JH, Dozois RR, Ilstrup D, van Heerden J (1990) The rela-tionship between pouchitis after pouch–anal anastomosis and extra-intestinal manifestations of chronic ulcerative colitis. Annals of Surgery 211: 622–9.

Lomont HA, De Petrillo AD, Sargeant EJ (1978) Psycho-sexual rehabilitation and exenterative surgery. Journal of Gynecological Oncology 6: 236–42.

Lynch H, Kunberling W, Albano J et al (1985) Hereditary non-polyposis colorectal cancer (Lynch syndromes I and II). Clinical description of resource. Cancer 56: 934–8.

McArdle CS, Hole D (1991) Impact of variability among surgeons on postoperative morbidity and mortality and ultimate survival (see comments). British Medical Journal 302(6791): 1501–5.

McDonald L, Anderson H (1984) Stigma in patients with rectal cancer – a community study. Journal of Epidemiology and Community Health 16: 284–90.

MacElveen-Hoenn P (1985) Sexual assessment and counselling. Seminars in Oncological Nursing L (1): 69–75.

McGonagle B (1988) A Patient Guide to the Surgery of Ulcerative Colitis: The Pelvic Pouch (Pull-through) Procedure. Cleveland, OH: Department of Colorectal Surgery, Cleveland Clinic Foundation.

McKenzie F (1988) Sexuality after total pelvic exenteration. Nursing Times 84(20): 27–30.

McLeod RS, Fazio VW (1984) Quality of life with continent ileostomy. World Journal of Surgery 8: 90–5.

McPheteridge L (1968) Nursing history: one means to personalised care. American Journal of Nursing 16: 68–75.

Malone D, McGrath F (1993) Optimising the detection of colorectal liver metastases with the Canadian health care system. Canadian Association of Radiology Journal 44: 5–13.

Maloney MJ (1995) Eating disorders during adolescence. Annales Nestle 53(3): 20–41.

Manworren RCB (1996) Developmental effects on the adolescent of a temporary ileostomy. Journal of Wound, Ostomy and Continence Nursing 23(4): 210–17.

Marcello PW, Roberts PL, Schoetz DJ, Coller JA, Murray JJ, Veidenheimer MC (1993) Long-term results of the ileoanal pouch procedure. Archives of Surgery 128: 500–4.

Martin LW, LeCoultre C, Shubert WK (1977) Total colectomy and mucosal proctectomy with preservation of continence in ulcerative colitis. Annals of Surgery 186(4): 477–80.

Maxwell R (undated) The ileo-anal pouch operation. Information sheet. Ileostomy Association of Great Britain and Ireland.

Medical Research Council Rectal Cancer Working Party (1996) Randomised trial of surgery alone versus radiotherapy followed by surgery for potentially operable locally advanced rectal cancer. Lancet 348: 1605–10.

Miles E (1908) A method of performing abdominoperineal excision for carcinoma of the rectum and of the terminal portion of the pelvic colon. Lancet 1812-13.

M'Koma AE (1994) Follow-up results of haematology data before and after restorative proctocolectomy: clinical outcome. Diseases of the Colon and Rectum 37: 932–7.

M'Koma AE, Lindquist K, Liljeqvist L (1994) Biochemical laboratory data in patients before and after restorative proctocolectomy. Annales de Chirurgie 48: 525–34.

Moertel C, Schutt A, Go V (1978) Carcinoembryonic antigen test for recurrent colorectal cancer. Journal of the American Medical Association 78: 1065–6.

Montgomery J (1997) Child consent. In Health Care Law. Oxford: Oxford University Press.

Morgado PJ, Wexner SD, James K, Nogueras JJ, Jagelman DG (1994) Ileal pouch–anal anastomosis: is preoperative anal manometry predictive of postoperative functional outcome? Diseases of the Colon and Rectum 37: 224–8.

Morson B (1985) Local excision for colorectal cancer: histological criterial for local excision. British Journal of Surgery (suppl.): S53-S54.

Mowschenson PM, Critchlow F (1995) Outcome of early surgical complications following ileoanal pouch operation without diverting ileostomy. The American Journal of Surgery 169: 143-5.

Mulgrew B, Dropkin M (1991) Coping with craniofacial resection. A case study. Head and Neck Cancer 4: 8–10.

Mullen P, Brehrens D, Chalmers T (1995) Barnett continent intestinal reservoir. Diseases of the Colon and Rectum 38: 573–82.

Murrary KF, Leichtner A (1997) Inflammatory bowel disease: treatment. International Seminars in Paediatric Gastroenterology and Nutrition 6(2): 7–10.

Muto T, Bussey H, Morson B (1975) The evolution of cancer of the colon and rectum. Cancer 36: 2251–70.

Nasmyth DG, Williams NS (1993) Pouch ecology. In Nicholls J, Bartolo D, Mortensen N (Eds) Restorative Proctocolectomy. Oxford: Blackwell Scientific.

Nasymth DG, Johnston D, Godwin PGR, Dixon MF, Smith A, Williams NS (1986) Factors influencing bowel function after ileal pouch–anal anastomosis. British Journal of Surgery 73: 469–73.

NAWCH (National Association for the Welfare of Children in Hospital) (1990) Setting Standards for Adolescents in Hospital. London: NAWCH.

Nemer FD, Rolstad BS (1985) The role of the ileoanal reservoir in patients with ulcerative colitis and familial polyposis. Journal of Enterostomal Therapy 12: 74–83.

Nicholls RJ, Harocopas C (1990) Ulcerative Colitis – a Guide for Patients. Ickenham: Convatec.

Nicholls R (1983) Proctocolectomy. l. Avoiding an ileostomy. Nursing Mirror (Feb 16): 46–7.

Nicholls RJ (1984) Restorative proctocolectomy with a 3 loop ileal reservoir for ulcerative colitis and familial adenomatous polyposis: clinical results in 66 patients followed for up to 6 years. Annals of Surgery 199: 383–8.

Nicholls RJ (1993) Controversies and practical problem solving. In Nicholls J, Bartolo D, Mortensen N (Eds) Restorative Proctocolectomy. Oxford: Blackwell Scientific.

Nicholls RJ, Lubowski DZ (1987) Restorative proctocolectomy: the four loop (W) reservoir. British Journal of Surgery 4: 564–6.

Nicholls R, Pezim M (1985) Restorative proctocolectomy with ileal reservoir for ulcerative colitis and familial polyposis coli. British Journal of Surgery 72: 470–4.

Nicholls RJ, Wells AD (1992) Undeterminate colitis. Baillière's Clinical Gastroenterology 6: 105–12.

Nicholls RJ, Belliveau P, Neill M, Wilks M, Tabaqchali S (1981b) Restorative proctocolectomy with ileal reservoir: a pathophysiological assessment. Gut 22: 462–8.

Nicholls S et al (1995) Linear growth after colectomy for ulcerative colitis in childhood. Journal of Paediatric Gastroenterology and Nutrition 21(1): 82–6.

Nicholls RJ, Lubowski DZ, Donaldson DR (1996) Comparison of colonic reservoir and straight colo-anal reconstruction after rectal excision. British Journal of Surgery 75: 318–20.

Nilsson LO, Andersson H, Hultèn L et al (1979) Absorption studies in patients six to ten years after construction of ileostomy reservoirs. Gut 20: 499–503.

Nilsson LO, Myrvold HE, Swolin B, Öjerskog B (1984) Vitamin B12 in plasma in patients with continent ileostomy and long observation time. Scandinavian Journal of Gastroenterology 19: 369–74.

Nordstrum G (1988) Urostomy patients – a strategy for care. Nursing Times 85(18): 32–4.

Northover JMA (1995) The use of prognostic markers in surgery for colorectal cancer. European Journal of Cancer 31a(7-8): 1207–9.

Norwich Pouch Support Group Member (1997) Roar! Issue no. 7: 9.

Oakley J (1991) Current thoughts on the aetiology and management of inflammatory bowel disease. World Council of Enterostomal Therapy Journal ll(2): 12–15.

O'Connell PR, Rankin DR, Weiland LH, Kelly KA (1986) Enteric bacteriology, absorption, morphology and emptying after ileal pouch–anal anastomosis. British Journal of Surgery 73: 909–14.

O'Connor B, Scott H, McLeod R, Blair J, Cohen Z (1998) Pregnancy, delivery and pouch function in females following the pelvic pouch procedure. ia Journal (159): 52–3.

Öjerskog B, Kock NG, Nilsson LO, Philipson BM, Ahrèn C (1990) Long-term follow-up of patients with continent ileostomies. Diseases of the Colon and Rectum 33: 184–9.

Oresland T (1996) Pelvic pouch or proctocolectomy and ileostomy? Eurostoma 14: (Summer): 4.2–4.3.

Orkin BA, Telander RL, Wolff BG, Perrault J, Ilstrup DM (1990) The surgical management of children with ulcerative colitis. The old vs. the new. Diseases of the Colon and Rectum 33(11): 947–55.

O'Sullivan M (1992) Quality of life after proctocolectomy and ileal pouch formation. Proceedings from the 9th Biennial Congress World Council of Enterostomal Therapists. Illinois: Hollister.

Padilla G, Grant M (1985) Quality of life as a cancer nursing outcome variable. Advances in Nursing Science (Oct): 45–60.

Panis Y, Poupard B, Nemeth J, Lavergne A, Hautefeuille P, Valleur P (1996) Ileal pouch–anal anastomosis for Crohn's disease. Lancet 347: 854–7.

Parker MC, Nicholls RJ (1992) Restorative proctocolectomy in patients after previous intestinal or anal surgery. Diseases of the Colon and Rectum 35: 681–4.

Parkin D, Muir C, Whelan S (1987) Cancer Incidence in Five Continents. Lyon: International Agency for Research on Cancer.

Parks A (1972) Transanal technique in low rectal anastomosis. Proceedings of the Royal Society of Medicine 65: 975–6.

Parks AG, Nicholls RJ (1978) Proctocolectomy without ileostomy for ulcerative colitis. British Medical Journal 2: 85–8.

Parsons R, Li GM, Rao M (1993) Hypermutability and mismatch repair deficiency in RER and tumour cells. Cell 75: 1227.

Pemberton JH (1993) Complications, management, failure and revisions. In Nicholls J, Bartolo D, Mortensen N (Eds) Restorative proctocolectomy. Oxford: Blackwell Scientific.

Pemberton JH, Kelly KA, Beaart RW, Dozois RR, Wolff BG, Ilstrup DM (1987) Ileal pouch–anal anastomosis for chronic ulcerative colitis. Long term results. Annals of Surgery 206: 504–13.

Pemberton J, Phillips S, Ready R, Zinsmeister A, Beahrs O (1989) Quality of life after Brook ileostomy and ileal pouch–anal anastomosis: comparison of performance status. Surgery 209(5): 1620–8.

Penna C et al (1993) Secondary proctectomy and ileal pouch–anal anastomosis after ileo-rectal anastomosis for familial adenomatous polyposis. British Journal of Surgery 80(12): 1621–3.

Pezim PE, Nicholls RJ (1985a) Restorative proctocolectomy with ileal reservoir for ulcerative colitis and familial adenomatous polyposis: a comparison of three reservoir designs. British Journal of Surgery 72: 470–4.

Pezim M, Nicholls R (1985b) Quality of life after restorative proctocolectomy with pelvic ileal reservoir. British Journal of Surgery 72(1): 31–3.

Phillips RKS et al (1983) Local recurrence after curative surgery for large bowel cancer – the overall picture. British Journal of Surgery 71: 12–16.

Phillips RKS (1991) Pelvic pouches. British Journal of Surgery 78: 1025.

Phillips RKS (1998) Ileal pouch–anal anastomosis for Crohn's disease. Gut 43: 303–8.

Phillips RKS, Spigelman AD, Thomson JPS (Eds) (1993) Familial Adenomatous Polyposis and Other Polyposis Syndromes. London: Edward Arnold.

Pincowsky D, Ekbom A (1995) Is there an increased risk of colorectal cancer among ulcerative colitis patients with primary sclerosing cholangitis? Gastroenterology 108: abstract 29.

Potter J (1996) Epidemilogic, environmental and lifestyle issues in coloretal cancer. Prevention and Early Detection of Colorectal Cancer. RAL Young. London: WB Saunders.

Potter J, Slattery M, Bostick R, Gapstur S (1993) Colon cancer: a review of the epidemiology. Epidemiological Review 15: 499–545.

Price B (1990) Body Image – Nursing Concepts and Care. London: Prentice Hall.

Price R (1993) How to make an assessment of altered body image in stoma patients. Eurostoma (4): 14.

Price R (1996) Illness careers: the chronic illness experience. Journal of Advanced Nursing 24: 275–9.

Pricolo VE, Potenti FM, Luks FI (1996) Selective preservation of the anal transition zone in ileoanal pouch procedure. Diseases of the Colon and Rectum 39: 871–7.

Primrose JN, Holdsworth PJ, Nasmyth DG, Womack N, Neal DE, Johnston D (1988) Intact anal sphincter with end to end ileoanal anastomosis for ulcerative colitis: comparison with mucosal proctectomy and pull-through anastomosis. British Journal of Surgery 74: 539.

Probert CSJ, Jayanthi V, Bhakta P, Wicks TCB, Mayberry JF (1993) How necessary is colectomy? An epidemiological study of the surgical management of ulcerative colitis amongst different ethnic groups in Leicestershire. European Journal of Gastroenterology and Hepatology 5: 17–20.

Quirke P, Durdey P, Dixon M, Williams N (1986) Local recurrence of rectal adenocarcinoma due to inadequate surgical resection. Lancet ii: 996–9.

Rafferty D (1995) Body image: using women who have had breast surgery as a case study. International Journal of Palliative Care 1(4): 195–9.

Ravitch MM, Sabiston DC (1947) Anal ileostomy with preservation of the sphincter. Surgery, Gynecology and Obstetrics 84: 1095–9.

Raymond JL, Becker JM (1986) Ileoanal pull-through: a new surgical alternative to ileostomy and a new challenge in diet therapy. Journal of the American Dietetic Association 86: 663–5.

Rintala RJ, Lindahl HG, Rasanen M (1997) Do children with repaired low anorectal malformations have normal bowel function? Journal of Paediatric Surgery 32(6): 823–6.

Rolstad B, Nemer F (1985) Management problems associated with ileoanal reservoir. Journal of Enterostomal Therapy 12(2): 41–8.

Rolstad B, Rothenberger D (undated) Ileo-anal Reservoir: A Patient Resource. Kalamazoo, MI: Upjohn.

Rolstad B, Wilson G, Volk-Tebbitt B (1985) Long term sexual status concerns in the client with ileostomy. Journal of Enterostomal Therapy 9(4): 10–12.

Romanos J, Stebbing JF, Mortensen NJ, Kettlewell MGW (1996) Restorative proctocolectomy in children and adolescents. Journal of Paediatric Surgery 31(12): 1655–8.

Rosenbaum TP, Shah PJR, Rose GA, Lloyd-Davis RW (1989) Cranberry juice helps the problem of mucus production in enterouroplasties. Neurology and Urodynamics 8(4): 344–5.

Rothenberger DA, Buls JG, Nivatvongs S, Goldberg SM (1985) The Park's S-ileal pouch–anal anastomosis after colectomy and mucosal proctectomy. American Journal of Surgery 149: 390–4.

Roussoux J, Fennerty L, Harlan W (1995) The evolution of the women's health initiative: a perspective from the NIH. American Women's Medical Association 50: 50–5.

Rutegard J, Ahsgren L, Janunger K (1988) Ulcerative colitis. Colorectal cancer risk in an unselected population. Annals of Surgery 208: 721–4.

Sagar PM, Lewis W, Holdsworth PJ, Johnston D, Micthell C, MacFie J (1993) Quality of life after restorative proctocolectomy with a pelvic reservoir compares favourably with that of patients with medically treated colitis. Diseases of the Colon and Rectum 36(6): 584–92.

Salemans JMJI, Nagengast FM (1995) Clinical and physiological aspects of ileal pouch–anal anastomosis. Scandinavian Journal of Gastroenterology 30(suppl. 212): 3–12.

Salemans JMJI, Nagengast FM, Tangerman A, Van Schaik A, De Haan AFJ, Jansen JBMJ (1993) Postprandial conjugated and unconjugated serum bile acid levels after proctocolectomy with ileal pouch–anal anastomosis. Scandinavian Journal of Gastroenterology 28: 786–90.

Salter M (1992a) What are the differences in body image between patients with a conventional stoma compared with those who have had a conventional stoma followed by a continent pouch? Journal of Advanced Nursing 17: 841–8.

Salter M (1992b) Aspects of sexuality for patients with stomas and continent pouches. Journal of Enterostomal Nursing 19: 126–30.

Salter M (1996) Advances in ileostomy care. Nursing Standard 11(9): 49–53.

Salter M (Ed) (1997) Altered Body Image - the Nurse's Role. London: Baillière Tindall.

Salter MJ (1988) Altered Body Image – the Nurse's Role. Chichester: John Wiley & Sons.

Santavirta J, Harmoinen A, Karvonen AL, Matikainen M (1991) Water and electrolyte balance after ileoanal anastomosis. Diseases of the Colon and Rectum 34: 115–18.

Saylor C, Yoder M (1988) Stigma. In Lubkin IM, Larsen PD (Eds) Chronic Illness: Impact and Interventions. Boston: Jones & Bartlett.

Schilder P (1935) The Image and the Appearance of the Human Body. Psyche Monographs No. 4. London: Kegan Paul, Trench, Truber.

Schjonsby et al (1977) Stagnant loop syndrome in patients with continent ileostomy. Gut 18: 795–9.

Scholefield J, Northover JMA (1995) Surgical management of rectal cancer. British Journal of Surgery 82: 745–8.

Scott AD, Phillips RKS (1989) Ileitis and pouchitis after colectomy for ulcerative colitis. British Journal of Surgery 76: 668–9.

Seidel SA, Peach SE, Newman M, Sharp KW (1999) Ileoanal pouch procedures: clinical outcomes and quality of life assessment. American Surgeon 65(1): 40–6.

Selby J, Friedman G, Quesenberry C, Weiss N (1992) A case control study of screening sigmoidoscopy and mortality from colo-rectal cancer. New England Journal of Medicine 326(10): 653–7.

Seow-Choen A, Tsunoda A, Nicholls RJ (1991) Prospective randomised trial comparing anal function after handsewn ileoanal anastomosis with mucosectomy versus stapled ileoanal anastomosis with mucosectomy in restorative proctocolectomy. British Journal of Surgery 78: 430–4.

Seow-Choen F (1993) Colonic pouch after low anterior resection of the distal third of the rectum. Annals of the Academy of Medicine, Singapore 22(2): 229–32.

Setti-Carraro PG, Talbot IC, Nicholls RJ (1998) Patterns of endoscopic and histological changes in the ileal reservoir after restorative proctocolectomy for ulcerative colitis. A long-term follow-up study. International Journal of Colorectal Disease 13(2): 103–7.

Setti-Carraro P, Talbot IC, Nicholls RJ (1994) Long-term appraisal of the histological appearances of the ileal reservoir mucosa after restorative proctocolectomy for ulcerative colitis. Gut 35: 1721–7.

Shamberger RC, Lillehei CW, Nurko S, Winter HS (1994) Anorectal function in children after ileo anal pull-through. Journal of Paediatric Surgery 29(2): 329–32.

Shamberger RC, Masek BJ, Leichtrei AM, Winter HS, Lillehei CW (1999) Quality of life assessment after ileoanal pull-through for ulcerative colitis and familial adenomatous polyposis. Journal of Paediatric Surgery 34(1): 163–6.

Sharp FR, Bell GA, Seal AM, Atkinson KG (1987) Investigations of the anal sphincter before and after restorative proctocolectomy. American Journal of Surgery 5153: 469–72.

Shelley H (1993) Adolescent needs in hospital. Paediatric Nursing 5(9): 16–18.

Shepherd NA (1989) Workshop pouchitis. International Journal of Colorectal Disease 4: 205–29.

Sidransky D, Tokino T, Hamilton S (1992) Identification of ras oncogene mutations in the stool of patients with curable colorectal tumours. Science 256: 102–5.

Simon J (1852) Ectopic vescicae (absence of the anterior walls of the bladder and pubic abdominal parietes): operation for directing the orifices of the ureters into the rectum: temporary success; subsequent death; autopsy. Lancet 2: 568–70.

Slade D (2000) The voice of experience. Journal of Wound, Ostomy and Continence Nursing 27: 201–6.

Slattery M, Abd-Elghany N, Kerbei R, Schumacher MC (1990) Physical activity and colon cancer: a comparison of various indicators of physical activity to evaluate the association. Epidemiology 1(6) 481–5.

Slors JFM, Ponson AE, Taat CW, Bosma A (1995) Risk of residual rectal mucosa after proctocolectomy and ileal pouch–anal reconstruction with the double-stapling technique. Diseases of the Colon and Rectum 38: 207–10.

Smith R (1984) Identity crisis. Nursing Mirror 158: 2–6.

Smitherman C (1981) Nursing Action for Health Promotion. London: FA Davis.

Spencer M, Barnett WO (1982) The continent ileal reservoir (Kock pouch): a new approach. Journal of Enterostomal Therapy 9: 8–13.

Stelzner M, Fonkalsrud EW, Buddington RK, Phillips JD, Diamond JM (1990) Adaptive changes in ileal mucosal nutrient transport following colectomy and endorectal ileal pull-through with ileal reservoir. Archives of Surgery 125: 586–90.

Stern H, Cohen Z, Wilson DR, Mickle DAG (1980) Urolithiasis risk factors in continent reservoir ileostomy patients. Diseases of the Colon and Rectum 23: 556–8.

Stewart J, Kumar D, Keighley MR (1994) Results of anal or low rectal anastomosis and pouch reconstruction for mega rectum and mega colon. British Journal of Surgery 81(7): 1051–3.

Stewart M (1986) Urinary diversion and bowel cancer. Annals of the Royal College of Surgeons of England 68: 98–102.

Stoddard F, Strand L, Murphy M (1992) Depression in children after recovery from severe burns. Journal of Burn Care Rehabilitation 13(3): 340–7.

Strader M (1989) The ileo-anal reservoir. Nursing Times 85(4): 48–50.

Swedish Rectal Cancer Group (1997) Improved survival with preoperative radiotherapy in rectal cancer. New England Journal of Medicine 336: 980–7.

Taylor TV, Bhandarkar DS, Seehra HK (1994) Quest for continence: surgery for ulcerative colitis and familial adenomatous polyposis. British Journal of Hospital Medicine 51(3): 108–10.

Telander RL et al (1981) Surgical treatment of ulcerative colitis in children. Surgery (Oct): 787–94.

Telander RL Spencer M, Perrault J, Telander D, Zingmeister AR (1990) Long term follow up of the ileoanal anastomosis in children and young adults. Surgery 108: 717–25.

Thompson-Fawcett MW, Jewell DP, Mortensen NJ (1997) Ileoanal reservoir dysfunction: a problem-solving approach. British Journal of Surgery 84(10): 1351–9.

Thompson-Fawcett MW, Mortensen NJ, Warren BF (1999) 'Cuffitis' and inflammatory changes in the columnar cuff, anal transitional zone and ileal reservoir after stapled pouch–anal anastomosis. Diseases of the Colon and Rectum 42: 348–55.

Tiainen J, Matikainen M (1999) Health-related quality of life after J-pouch–anal anastomosis for ulcerative colitis: long-term results. Scandinavian Journal of Gastroenterology 36(4): 601–5.

Tuckson WB, Fazio VW (1991) Functional comparison between double and triple ileal loop pouches. Diseases of the Colon and Rectum 34: 17–21.

Turner B (1992) Regulating Bodies: Essays in Medical Sociology. London: Routledge.

Tyus FJ, Austhof SI, Chima CS, Keating C (1992) Diet tolerance and stool frequency in patients with ileoanal reservoirs. Journal of the American Dietetic Association 92: 861–3.

Utsunomiya AJJ, Iwana T, Imago M et al (1980) Total colectomy, muscosal proctectomy and ileoanal anastomosis. Diseases of the Colon and Rectum 23: 459–66.

Valiente MA, Bacon HE (1955) Construction of pouch using 'pantaloon' technique for pull-through following total colectomy. American Journal of Surgery 90: 6621–43.

Verne J and others (1996) A population based randomised study comparing uptake and yield of flexible sigmoidoscopy screening with Haemoccult. British Medical Journal 317: 182–5.

Virgo K and others (1995) Cost of patient follow-up after potentially curative colorectal cancer treatment. Journal of the American Medical Association 273: 1837–41.

Wade B (1989) The plight of the patient with a temporary stoma. Senior Nurse 9(4): 27–9.

Waldron RI, Donovan J, Drumm J, Mottram S, Tedman S (1995) Emergency presentation and mortality from colorectal cancer in the elderly. British Journal of Surgery 73: 216–20.

Wallace E (1993) Nursing a teenager with burns. British Journal of Nursing 2(5): 278–81.

Walls S (1997) Why getting better can be a scary experience. Roar! Issue no. 7: 4–5.

Wammeck R, Fisch M, Hohenfellner R (1995) Ureterosigmoidostomy and the Mainz Pouch II. In Webster GD, Goldwasser B (Ed) Urinary Diversion: Scientific Foundations and Clinical Practice. Oxford: Isis Medical Media.

Wassner A (1982) The impact of mutilating surgery or trauma on body image. International Nursing Review 29(3): 86–90.

Webb C (1984) Nurses' knowledge and attitudes about sexuality: report of a study. Nursing Education Today 7: 209–14.

Webb C, O'Neill J (1989) Nurse's attitudes about sexuality in health care. A review of the literature. Nursing Education Today 7: 75–87.

Weinryb R, Gustavsson J, Liljeqvist L et al (1995) A prospective study of the quality of life after pelvic pouch operation. Journal of American College of Surgeons 180: 589–95.

Wells R (1990) Sexuality: an unknown word for patients with a stoma. In Senn, H, Glaus J (Eds) Results in Cancer Research. Berlin: Springer-Verlag.

Wendland B (1996) Nutrition matters for pouch patients. Quarterly Journal of the Ileostomy and Internal Pouch Support Group 150: 17.

Wexner SD, Jensen L, Rothenberger DA, Wong WD, Goldberg SM (1989) Long-term functional analysis of the ileoanal reservoir. Diseases of the Colon and Rectum 32: 275–81.

Whiteway J, Nicholls RJ, Morson B (1985) The role of surgical local excision in the treatment of rectal cancer. British Journal of Surgery 72: 694–7.

Williams JM (1998) What pre-operative expectations do ileo-anal pouch patients have of their surgery, post-operative nursing and lifestyle following surgery. Unpublished BSc thesis, Royal College of Nursing, affiliated to Manchester University.

Williams N (1986) An alternative to an ileostomy? Ileostomy Journal 153: 10–13.

Williams N, Durdy P, Johnston D (1985) The outcome following sphincter-saving resection and abdominoperineal resection for low rectal cancer. British Journal of Surgery 72: 595–8.

Winawer S, Fletcher RH, Miller L (1997) Colorectal cancer screening: clinical guidelines and rationale. Gastroenterolgy 112: 594–642.

Wood S (1996) Nutrition and the short bowel syndrome. In Myers C (Ed) Stoma Care Nursing - A Patient-centred Approach. London: Arnold.

Woodhouse CRJ (1994) The Infective Metabolic and Histological Consequences of Enterocystoplasty. European Board of Urology European Urology Update Series, Vol. 3. Union Européanne des Médécins Specialistes.

Woodhouse CRJ, Christofides M (1998) Modified ureterosigmoidostomy (Mainz II) technique and early results. British Journal of Urology 81: 247-52.

Woodhouse CRJ, Gordon EM (1994) The Mitrofanoff principle for urethral failure. British Journal of Urology 73: 55–60.

Ziv Y, Church JM, Oakley JR, McGannon E, Fazio VW (1995) Surgery for the teenager with familial adenomatous polyposis ileo-rectal anastomosis or restorative proctocolectomy. International Journal of Colorectal Disease 10(1): 6–9.

Further reading

Bellinger MF (1989) The history of urinary diversion and undiversion. Journal of Enterostomal Therapy 16(1): 39–46.

Bussey HJR (1975) F.A.P. Baltimore: John Hopkins University Press.

Forbes A (1997) Clinicians' Guide to Inflammatory Bowel Disease. London: Chapman & Hall.

Mitrofanoff P (1980) Cystomies continente trans-appendiculaire dans le traitment des vessies neurologiques. Chirurgie Pediatrique 2111: 297–307.

Phillips RKS, Spigelman AD, Thomson JPS (1987) F.A.P. and Other Polyposis Syndromes. London: Edward Arnold.

Wagstaff KE, Woodhouse CRJ, Rose GA, Duffy PG, Ransley PG (1991) Blood and urine analysis in patients with intestinal bladders. Journal of Urology 68: 311–16.

Woodhouse CRJ (1991) The Mitrofanoff principle for continent urinary diversion. World Council of Enterostomal Therapists Journal 11(1): 12–15.

Index